Possibilities
with
Parkinson's

A Fresh Look and Collection of Essays on the
Journey of Discovery

Possibilities
with
Parkinson's

A Fresh Look and Collection of Essays on the
Journey of Discovery

By Dr. C.

atmosphere press

Published by Atmosphere Press

Cover design by Kevin Stone

"Changes," words and music by Phil Ochs, copyright © 1965 Barricade Music, Inc. All rights controlled and administered by Almo Music Corp. Reprinted by Permission of Hal Leonard LLC.

atmospherepress.com

Why This Book Was Written

The Parkinson's Foundation in 2018 published their study on the prevalence of Parkinson's Disease: 5 Facts You Should Know About the Study:[1]

1) The 2018 Prevalence Project estimate draws from large and diverse populations.
2) The new study estimate is nearly double the 1978 study prevalence number.
3) By 2020, 930,000 people in the US will be living with Parkinson's. This number will rise to 1.2 million by 2030.
4) The new study confirms that men are more likely to have Parkinson's disease (PD) than women and that the number of those diagnosed with PD increases with age, regardless of sex.
5) The new study found that the prevalence of people diagnosed with PD varies by region. Study researchers will devote more time to find out how.

I have Parkinson's disease. I am one of those 930,000 people in the US with this condition.

This book shares the story of one patient questioning the current precepts of Parkinson's disease, (often referred to as "PD" by clinicians and patients alike and will be referred to in that manner in this book) and developing a new theory describing Parkinson's disease. The theory is the result of reading scientifically published material, reaching out to medical professionals, listening to what other PD patients express as their concerns, hopes, fears and frustrations, and analyzing my own progression with the disease. The author's background as a scientific theoretician combined with clinical experience focused on recovery from brain trauma provides a

---

[1] Parkinson's Foundation Prevalence Project Finds Number of People With Parkinson's Severely Underestimated. Published on Parkinsons.org

unique perspective on living with PD.

The story presented here is bound within the biases of the author. My story is presented not as puffery but as a scientific journey by a research scientist who also has an unusual form of Parkinson's disease. The story is presented not for ego gratification but as a medium for communicating complex scientific issues to the general population, specifically those affected by Parkinson's disease. If the new scientific information contained within this book is to be useful, then it should be communicated to all those who need it. The combination of story, science, and inspiration is a format we sought to put in every essay to make the information accessible to all on different levels.

So much is changing in the world of Parkinson's. Hundreds of papers are published every month. New discoveries are being researched, and new patients are stepping forward with their diagnoses, symptoms, and questions. Disheartening is that much of the medical community still relies upon the 200-year-old medical description of Parkinson's disease as a neurological syndrome, which was first presented in 1817 by James Parkinson. As more is discovered about this disease, more questions arise. One cannot help but imagine if other chronic diseases, or cancer, were restricted to antiquated theories of presentation, diagnosis, and treatment, whether those outdated answers would be satisfactory to patient communities. Hopefully, this book will nudge PD providers to take a fresh look at how they view the disease.

This book is about possibility and about finding hope for better outcomes when facing chronic illness, in particular Parkinson's disease. It's a story about one man's quest to find scientifically sound information to guide the development of a brain therapy that could make living with Parkinson's disease a little easier. This quest led to the development of a new theory describing why Parkinson's disease has such a diverse presentation in the general population. This theory is presented at the end of the book. If you're like some mystery novel readers who need to read the end of the story first, <u>don't do it</u>. The book describes the genuine struggle to discover this new theory and to live better with a chronic disease. It is a struggle of finding meaning and purpose in the midst of pain and suffering. The journey contains many useful tips on how to live well with PD, and each one is tried and tested by the author, who states, "If I can't walk it, then I won't talk it."

These 100 essays shared here were first published on the website Parkinson's News Today by BioNews Services, an online medical news service emphasizing the patient's voice as an integral part of living better with chronic illness.[2] The columns began in August 2018 and continue weekly. The new Spectrum Stage Theory for Parkinson's can be found in the last eight essays, but the road to its discovery is just as beautiful. The essays intersperse the "heavy" science with the author's experiences, written in a lighter note and hopefully relatable to the reader's own life.

"Conversations with Neo"[3] began in August 2019. "Neo" has become a way to present complex information in a

---

[2] BioNews Today holds the values that "We bring awareness and help give a voice to those in the rare disease community. We work to build opportunities for people to access information freely, in an easy to understand way, and which helps them experience life as they choose. We have structured our organization in a style that encourages the involvement of our audience." I have been honored and blessed to share my thoughts and research on their website which can be found at https://parkinsonsnewstoday.com/

[3] "Neo" represents the processes of the neocortex in the brain. The neocortex is part of the **cerebral cortex**. It is involved in higher functions such as sensory perception, generation of **motor** commands, spatial reasoning, conscious thought, and in humans, language. In my writing, "Neo" provides the perfect foil for questioning my logical processes. He has become a character of his own, asking questions that readers would ask, or that I ask myself.

personable format. Neo has become a favorite character among readers. He reflects the conversations we all have with ourselves in those moments of quiet contemplation or screaming frustration. PD can be difficult to understand, and not understanding what is happening just makes everything worse.

"Dr. C." is not a medical doctor. He writes from his clinical expertise with a Ph.D. rehabilitation counseling specializing in brain trauma recovery, and from personal experiences with the disease. References are cited, using footnotes, throughout the essays to direct readers to the sources of information used. Effort was made to use primary sources from reputable websites, organizations, and peer-reviewed scientific and medical reports. The references also refer to essays on Parkinson's News Today, published by BioNews. The writings focus on identifying techniques and strategies that support the PD patient who wants to continue with the highest quality of life possible, accept and manage the challenges of the disease, and realize that they are not alone in their feelings and experiences. Much medical research is being directed to this disease, and readers are encouraged to consult with their medical provider before trying any of the ideas presented here.

Each essay in the book was written to be a stand-alone document. The reader can pick up this book at any time, read one essay, put the book down, reflect on the essay, and return to read more later. The new theory is built upon the foundation of information in a dozen essays leading to the theory, particularly in the second half of the book. New ideas require a foundation of information prior to presenting the new idea. This happens in many places throughout the book, but is most obvious with the new theory presented at the end of the book. The new theory is built upon the foundation of information in a dozen essays leading to the theory. Bringing this useful information together into one book, rather than scattered among separate Internet pages, should make it easier for readers to both access and follow. In addition, as a response to readers' comments to the columns, clarification notes have been added to the end of some of the short essays.

The story of finding a new theory and opening the door to more possibilities for Parkinson's disease is presented as a collection of short essays. Originally, these essays were published online at www.ParkinsonsNewstoday.com. Although we – "Mrs. Dr. C.," the editors, and "Dr. C." – have made some tweaks to these essays to enhance readability of the book, as a whole we have not changed the original intent of the 100 essays that led up to the publishing of the new theory. We have added a longer essay at the end of the book as an epilogue of hope for the future.

In the history of science, sometimes people with the right talents are put in the right circumstances where they can make a difference. Dr. C.'s life is unique in the combination of life events, education, training, and a personal relationship with the disease. His tour of duty in the Marines exposed him to agent orange toxins, which resulted in Parkinson's disease, but his military experience also provided knowledge about how far one can push oneself to reach a goal. Dr. C. used this knowledge many times as he earned four a Bachelor's degree, two Master's degrees and a Doctorate which represent academic training in both research science and counseling/therapy. During the past 60 years, Dr. C. has been trained as both a theoretician and a hands-on brain rehabilitation therapist. This dual approach of theory and brain rehabilitation is reflected throughout the essays.

A special note of recognition and gratitude to our first-line editor Robin Ketchen; the BioNews columns and editor teams, especially Brad Dell, Matt LaFleur, Dave Boddiger, Paige Wyant; my family and friends; the New London and Concord Parkinson's Support Groups; and all those readers of my Parkinson's News Today column whose comments encourage

Introduction: About the Authors

Most books don't include much beyond a brief biography for the authors. "Married, kids, and lives in Wherever" is about the limit of self-reveal. In our cases, however, we are two lives that have taken on the challenges that a chronic illness or disease, like Parkinson's, poses. We are not alone.

We are a husband-and-wife team. We came from quite different backgrounds in our family socioeconomic experiences. Beyond that disparity, however, is a true melding of complementary skills and personalities, joined in many common interests and dedication to being the best we can each strive to be and supporting our partner to do so as well. Combining these pieces into a sustainable marriage has given us "Dr. C." and "Mrs. Dr. C." We prefer writing under these pseudonyms as our lives are being revealed to many readers. It gives us a little distance and some literary license from our true identities and allows us the ability to share more intimate events.

We both had military experiences. Mrs. Dr. C. was the daughter of a career non-commissioned officer in the US Air Force. Dr. C. signed up for the Vietnam war effort because he needed a way to afford higher education. The exposures during his brief military service have impacted both our lives. Dr. C. deals with the physical repercussions of toxic exposure. Mrs. Dr. C. is steadfast and diligent in making sure the eligibility requirements for Veteran's Administration benefits and services are followed, the forms are complete, and the files document everything, not to mention all the driving to and from various VA facilities. The impact of both Dr. C's service-connected disabilities profoundly impacts Mrs. Dr. C. as a wife and now a caregiver. Our writing often includes Mrs. Dr. C.'s frustrations and perspectives that probably many family members of patients with PD experience.

With a bachelor's degree in geology and education from the University of Vermont, and a master's from Dartmouth in geology, Dr. C. was going to be a high school science teacher. But life took some strange twists and he ended up working as a theoretician in mineral deposits for an Atlantic Richfield subsidiary for 8 years. In the mid-1980s, the mineral, oil, and gas industry took a big hit and jobs were eliminated worldwide. It was at this point that we decided that returning to an educational profession was his career move. He started with substitute teaching and then moved into clinical rehabilitation with a master's in counseling from the University of New Hampshire. He continued with clinical work for 10 years, but decided that graduate-level education was where he could make the most impact. So, he went back to school after the younger of our two children graduated high school... and successfully completed a Ph.D. program at Syracuse University in rehabilitation counseling. His emphasis in clinical work was brain trauma, and with his Ph.D., he explored the counseling relationship with patients. Shortly after receiving his Ph.D., he was hired as an adjunct professor in health and human services at a small private college in Vermont and was advanced to assistant professor during his 10-year tenure. Never in our wildest dreams did we anticipate how this road in life would lead us to writing a book from a patient perspective.

Mrs. Dr. C. had 45 years in health care, mostly administrative and IT support. She always tells our medical providers that "I'm your worst nightmare because I know what all those 'big words' mean." Between the two of us, any new medical diagnosis is worth understanding. We research the genesis of any major symptoms, educating ourselves on treatment options, and attempt to assimilate that knowledge into self-care treatment plans that align with the professional medical community. One of our hallmarks of this book, and the essays on BioNews Today, is to provide readers with links to medical information. We review many, and select what we think are the best to share. The footnotes throughout this book are provided to offer these resources to our readers.

It hasn't been easy. We, like so many people, have had "good" providers and "bad" providers. The "bad" ones aren't lacking in medical skills – they lack in being able to understand the patient's perspective. They jump to conclusions or don't read what has been clearly documented in previous tests and evaluations. They are an inevitable hurdle that many patients face. And providers are confronted by us when we are not willing to simply accept their shortcomings. In essence, proactive and educated patients are often not the people providers want in their medical exam rooms. One telling comment, given by a family practitioner to Mrs. Dr. C. when she expressed grave concerns about foot-dragging, fatigue that would last for days, and other early neuromuscular symptoms, was the following: "I don't know what your husband has, but you better be able to support the family because he isn't going to be able to much longer." That was 15 years before the "official" Parkinson's diagnosis. We made our own efforts to accommodate the growing disability – seeking out flexible employment, being aware of the "bad" days, and adjusting schedules for what quickly became the endless round of evaluations to get treatment.

In 2002, Dr. C. was diagnosed with an eye condition that eventually was recognized by the Veterans Administration as service-connected. During evaluation, there were additional eye conditions that suggested to us that perhaps he was showing early signs of Parkinson's. It took us several years to find a VA neurologist who agreed. The biggest challenge since 2000 has been that most neurologists tend to look at the "classic" Parkinson's patient for overt and dramatic symptoms.

Dr. C. doesn't have a tremor but matches up with almost all the other symptoms that are generally overlooked by neurologists. He was not satisfied that his disease process was being ignored by other neurologists, and felt that many Parkinson's patients who fall short of the tremulous shaking symptoms but experience good relief with PD medications were being underserved. Having been a research scientist, a brain rehab clinician, a theoretician, and now a patient, we felt we were in a good position to start writing about our experiences as the disease unfolds and progresses.

The "double whammy" with the eye condition has left him legally blind now. There is no cure and only treatment when the retina appears to be on the verge of rupture. A couple of providers missed the early signs, and he has had three ruptures – another example of adverse outcomes when providers do not listen to patients. He has ongoing medical surveillance to try to tamp down the possibility of more vision loss, but there is no guarantee that he will not lose the remaining vision at some point. His Parkinson's is slowly progressing. We moved this year out of New England because the winter conditions there were making it very unsafe for both of us and treatment at the VA required a four- or five-hour drive one way (in good weather). We have relocated to a warmer climate, closer to family, and he is receiving particularly good treatment with only an hour's drive to a major VA center. Still, it's been a year of upheaval, selling our old house within 24 hours of listing it, moving through early stages of the COVID-19 pandemic in April, upgrading and renovating a 50-year-old house for ADA safety, and then trying to find some mental and psychological equilibrium after all of that.

We also want to take a moment to thank the Veteran's Administration and the staff who serve every day to meet the ongoing medical conditions many veterans have. It is our honor to say some of the best providers have made a difference in how we face both Parkinson's and the vision loss. We salute their efforts and say, "thank you for your service."

The essays include discussion about having a second chronic condition. Many PD patients, particularly those in the elder years, face other chronic medical issues. We are at that age in our lives where many family and friends are facing severe non-PD medical issues. No one else in the family has PD, but we are acutely aware that many "elders" face serious diseases. PD symptoms may limit how other medical conditions are handled, so it becomes a balancing act to manage multiple issues. In Dr. C.'s case, the loss of vision impacts how he coordinates hand movements. PD patients can lose the fine motor control to write with a pen, cook on a stove, and navigate stairs or curbs. Add to those challenges the inability to see the pen on the paper, find the correct controls on the stove (or need to replace the controls with safer digital appliances), or have the partner walk closely to identify "curb ahead" or "mind the gap" to avoid obstacles.

For several years, we managed to post one essay a week on Parkinson's News Today, except for holiday weeks. Dr. C. starts with the general theory and ideas, Mrs. Dr. C. does much of the research for scientific and medical information, then we write several versions before sending to a proofreader and submitting to the editors at BioNews. The columns are published under "Dr. C." as his clinical background could very easily suggest to readers that he would be able to give medical advice. He does not. Our intent is to share scientific and medical information on the research and treatment being done for Parkinson's. We have incorporated a more friendly "blog" writing style to be reader-friendly and to give information that is without the "heavy" medical and scientific information we read. It also gives us an opportunity to put a personal story in that shares the fear, frustrations, occasional successes of life's challenges with this disease.

Last year, we asked BioNews if they could determine the number of page views that a few columns generated. We weren't sure what to expect. There is a mechanism for readers to comment on articles, and we steadfastly respond to the readers. Seems only right – if we can suggest further reading, we do. Sometimes, we just acknowledge their lives, or encourage them to keep trying – and we always, always, thank them for taking the time to read the columns. To get an idea of how the columns were being received, we asked BioNews to see if they could determine the number of "hits" or "reads." To our amazement, several columns we picked for review had between 10,000 and 15,000 "hits" – one exceeded 45,000. We have received comments from Europe, Australia, India, and many different locations in the US. At this point, we decided, with the support of BioNews, to consolidate the essays into a book. Having both been avid readers, we appreciate the concept of a print or eBook format for readers. Moving back and forth through ideas seems much easier with book in hand rather than sitting in front of the PC. We are so incredibly grateful for BioNews in their continued support and contract renewals that we will continue with them. But the idea of a book is very intriguing for us.

So here we are. We continue to reach out and write columns. We appreciate that you, the reader, have taken the time to be interested in this book. As always, to all our readers, we thank you. We hope that you find some information, inspiration, and a connection to both of us.

Table of Contents

Table of Illustrations

"Changes"

Sit by my side, come as close as the air,
Share in a memory of gray;
Wander in my words, dream about the pictures
That I play of changes.
Green leaves of summer turn red in the fall
To brown and to yellow they fade.
And then they have to die, trapped within
the circle time parade of changes.

Scenes of my young years were warm in my mind,
Visions of shadows that shine.
'Til one day I returned and found they were the
Victims of the vines of changes.
The world's spinning madly, it drifts in the dark
Swings through a hollow of haze,
A race around the stars, a journey through
The universe ablaze with changes.

Moments of magic will glow in the night
All fears of the forest are gone
But when the morning breaks they're swept away by
golden drops of dawn, of changes.
Passions will part to a strange melody.
As fires will sometimes burn cold.
Like petals in the wind, we're puppets to the silver
strings of souls, of changes.

Your tears will be trembling, now we're somewhere else,
One last cup of wine we will pour
And I'll kiss you one more time, and leave you on
the rolling river shores of changes.

~ Phil Ochs (1966)

One Man's Quest to Live Well with PD

This is my story about living well with a chronic disease, so before I delve into the diverse range of topics presented, let me introduce myself to you. I was diagnosed with Parkinson's disease (PD) in my early 60s. It is an idiopathic form, and thus harder for others to see. I feel the symptoms of rigidity, inaccurate muscle aiming, slowing of movement and exaggerated emotions. There are other symptoms in various body parts – GI, urinary, eyes – that medical research has identified as being associated with, or caused by, PD. Providers from these specialties have ruled out other causes and seem to accept, grudgingly, that PD is at play throughout my body. At this stage, I have a very faint tremor. My handwriting is getting almost illegible, so I use the computer extensively. Another medical condition is now limiting my ability to see, so that impacts my balance and walking – moving through the "space-time continuum," as Mrs. Dr. C. puts it. I have a good response to Sinemet, extremely limited response to pain/muscle relaxant medications in general, and still experience a slow but relentless progression in my symptoms.

Over the past several years, additional PD-related symptoms have emerged. Symptoms that are not confirmed by other medical processes (or "aging" – that favorite fallback by many practitioners when no apparent anomaly is easily identified as a causative factor) can be discovered in the "also included" list of most PD patients' experiences[4]. These additional manifestations (often referred to as "non-motor symptoms") are making their way into the awareness of the medical community. I can see their effects daily and I am committed to making sense of what is happening and to attaining the highest quality of life in the face of PD symptoms. These essays will share this journey and insights gained along the way.

I am also a researcher and writer (see www.DrC.life) and after years of hearing, "You look great, I don't see the PD in you," while having the worst of the symptoms under control through medication, I thought it was time to put pen to paper. I have a unique background that combines clinical experience helping people with a background as a research scientist and teacher – which means that I have the ability to reframe things so that they may be viewed in a new light.

In these essays, there will be new ideas you might not have heard before, and they will be mostly ideas that are reframed – a fresh look. In every discussion, I have tried to validate through published scientific or medical journals rather than solely relying upon anecdotal patient experiences. The patient experiences are not to be dismissed, but serve as a starting point for discussion. Often these recountings of symptoms in the columns have generated reader comments that "I experience that also!" These writings represent my struggle to make meaning out of Parkinson's disease and what it is doing to my life.

The unique perspective that these essays bring to discussions about attaining a quality of life with Parkinson's disease is one I believe will be of interest to the reader. I have a Ph.D. in rehabilitation counseling specialized in treatment of cerebral-neurological disorders. I developed rehabilitation

---

[4] Parkinson's Foundation. Understanding Parkinson's, Non-Motor Symptoms. Online at www.Parkinsons.org

plans for people to attain a higher quality of life after terrible things had happened to their brains. I am also a scientist, and over the last five years, have done extensive research on what would be the ideal rehabilitation plan for a person like me with early signs of PD. I have put such a plan in place for my own life (though not as perfect as I would like, as I struggle with my own recommendations, like cutting back on ice cream!).

In my opinion, tackling the disease head-on with a vigorous rehabilitation plan makes as much a difference in the quality of my life as medication. I can't replace the medications, but I do not rely solely upon their effect without a holistic approach. My personal plan and weekly goals are 15 to 20 hours of exercise, 15 to 20 hours of mental stimulation activities, an ADA house, living close to support from family, decreased stress, healthy diet and doing things that are fun. That's the basics of the plan. There are good days and bad days, as every PD patient knows, so my plan must be flexible. The hours often get skewed from one goal to another. I get frustrated when I can't get outside to exercise, or my eyes can't focus on the computer. There is a lot of fine-tuning that happens when the basic plan is applied specifically to the needs of one person, like you, the reader.

Any rehabilitation plan needs to consider where a person falls within the spectrum of Parkinson's symptoms, where they are physically, mentally, and psychologically in their lives, and what their goals for healthy living are. Hopefully, this book will help the reader to make sense of the wide diversity of symptoms that befall patients with PD, put a personalized rehab plan in place, and live better with the disease.

This book is personal, but in every essay I try to leave reader with something that might improve the quality of their life with Parkinson's. It is a journey seeking to attain and maintain a high quality of life in the face of difficult brain changes. It is a journey we will take together.

A Preliminary Look at the Parkinson's Disease Spectrum

The needs of PD patients are quite varied. You may have read about the large symptom diversity in the PD population. It may be thought of as a spectrum, where some people display little or no symptoms of a certain type, and others describe that same symptom as severe. It is a spectrum which has yet to be well defined. It is a conundrum that plagues providers when the disease presents so differently among patients. If measured or at least formally considered in a clinical evaluation, several parameters in this spectrum could help us to gain more understanding of PD.

I have sat in support groups and given presentations to PD patients. Some show the obvious shaking symptoms. Others do not exhibit any symptoms at all. One sees the photos used in medical promotional materials of smiling, happy, engaged Parkinson's patients. One can't help but wonder, "Is that me?" "Is that what I could be?" "Is that how others see me?"

Clinical professionals have, to this point, divided the disease into the "shaking type" and the "rigid akinetic type." Patients range in severity of symptoms in each of the two types. It is likely that these two types fall on a spectrum of symptom manifestation with shaking and rigidity at opposite ends merging to overlap each other in most patients. Let's call these Parameter One: Tremors, and Parameter Two: Rigidity.

Some PD patients also have autonomic muscle involvement, e.g., reduced blinking, urinary flow issues or sexual dysfunction, and bowel movement problems. This can be considered Parameter Three: Decreased functioning of autonomic muscles.

Patients also fall on a spectrum of decline in both cognitive function and emotive control (Parameters Four and Five). Not to make the whole thing overly complicated, but two more

Parameters (Six and Seven) need to be added to paint a decent portrait of the PD spectrum – patient history (pre-Parkinson's brain and motor/nerve activity) and their current and past rehabilitation and treatment plan.

Here are the seven parameters possibly governing the spectrum of PD presentation in patients:

1) Shaking symptoms (fine and gross motor) and associated pain/fatigue.
2) Rigid symptoms (fine and gross motor) and associated pain/fatigue.
3) Involuntary muscle (referred to as "non-motor" changes – usually hidden in presentation to others.
4) Decreased cognitive performance, sometimes clearly evident, other times masked by age-related status.
5) Emotional control changes.
6) Premorbid history – what was this brain used for? (Includes nervous system history, medical history, previous mental capabilities or skills, exercise history.)
7) Current and past rehabilitation plan and treatment.

I think all Parkinson's patients should be evaluated using these seven parameters. If we could hold in our minds these seven parameters and see that they contain the potential for a wide-spectrum landscape of PD diversity, then it may be possible to improve the quality of life for many of those afflicted with PD.

There are obstacles to painting a PD landscape with these seven parameters and having results with enough detail to be of clinical value. The first obstacle is the ability to measure the changes that take place in PD patients along the seven parameters across the stages of the disease development – from early to late manifestations. Thus far, our technology, and our clinical senses, have not been successful at clarifying the spectrum during the early years of PD.

The second obstacle is linked to the ability of the medical practitioner to gather, access, and synthesize material necessary for painting the PD spectral landscape using the seven parameters. Medical education often falls back to the "tried and true" theories that have held ground for over 200 years. Rotating through different providers in a teaching hospital makes for a tedious retelling of one's life and symptoms. Sometimes, the provider just sees me on that "good day" and not the "bad day" and that is their only frame of reference. Staying current with new research is time-consuming and time is often the biggest management challenge for a practitioner. The landscape needs not only to be painted for thousands of PD patients, but it also needs to be painted with enough specific clarity so that an individual patient sitting with the practitioner can clearly be shown his/her special place in the spectrum.

A New Look at Freezing: Scenario Looping Breakdown as an Early Symptom

We have examined the idea of PD patients exhibiting symptoms on a spectrum. What can help with the finer details of understanding this spectrum are both technological and scientific breakthroughs that measure the prominent presenting features of PD. One such presenting feature of PD that needs more examination is the movement feature called "freezing." I am proposing here that there is an early PD symptom variation of freezing, called *scenario looping breakdown*.

When I first heard the term "freezing," I pictured a deer frozen in the headlights of a car. That wide-eyed stare as the car headed in their direction may not have registered as a threat until it was too late. It wasn't until I started experiencing subtle variations of not being able to move a given muscle (it was "frozen," totally unresponsive to my mental commands) that I understood freezing was connected to something I found when I was working with people who had neurological impairments. At that time, I called it *scenario looping.*

Arriving at the answer involves "looping" through the scenario, over and over, weighing the consequences of any action, until you arrive at a satisfactory answer of what action to take. Scenarios of all types are presented to us every day. We are always faced with decisions about how to use our time, how to structure our language, and even how to structure our internal dialog. All of this is connected to scenario looping.

Scenario looping is also connected to motor sequencing. You need to tell your body to do the necessary motor sequences. We may not think of motor sequences as part of how we interact with the day because so much of our movement, like walking, is nearly automatic. We have done so much walking in our lives that it has become a motor sequence we don't think about – an overlearned motor scenario loop. It can run on "autopilot" – a small string of actions that can function in the background of your mind almost automatically. While it is functioning properly, you can simultaneously have a conversation or listen to music or sing along with the music. Despite the saying, "you can walk and chew gum at the same time," if you have PD, you can't.

It is possible that scenario looping breakdowns are symptoms indicating the presence of PD. Here is an example: I just finished making a PB&J sandwich, and I want to put the peanut butter jar back in the cupboard. Now I have the sandwich on a plate and the plate is in my left hand, the jar of peanut butter is in my right hand, but the top to the jar is on the counter. I want to put the PB away, but for a moment I freeze, staring at the lid of the PB jar on the counter. The motor steps should happen almost without thought. Put down the plate, grab the lid, screw it on, and put the peanut butter jar away. It is motor sequencing, scenario looping through the choices that need to be made to complete the task and arrive at the desired outcome. But it takes me a few moments to think what the sequence of actions should be to accomplish the task. I shouldn't have to think so hard to do this! Coordinating my muscles to not drop the entire collection of jar, plate, and sandwich is the additional challenge.

The new term scenario looping breakdown is reframing the occurrence of the PD freezing feature in hopes that early PD symptoms might be more easily diagnosed.

Note: There are additional essays that address this specific breakdown associated with PD:

- Oh, What a Drag it Is! Foot Problems as an Early Sign
- Taking a Careful Look at Apathy – It Could Be Motor Hesitation
- Movement Fluidity Improves within Formal Settings
- Rethinking Exercise
- Let's Face It – Mindful Mouth Movements

As the disease progresses, I am finding that constant attention to mindful movements is important – particularly when asking my body to go from one position to another position, for example, getting out of a chair and walking, or abruptly changing direction while walking. Because of the breakdown in scenario looping, the autopilot that I have relied upon does not work well. I will think, "I'm going to go to the kitchen and get a snack." If I do this automatically, without being mindful of my movements, then almost invariably my body will stumble because it is not automatically engaging in the process of movement. I think one of the reasons I have encountered so few falls thus far in my life with PD is because of my concerted effort to practice mindful movements. But there were two rather dramatic falls in my experiences that really brought this problem to light. Both times I was otherwise engaged in thinking about something unrelated to the hazards that lay before me.

Deep Fatigue – More than Just Being Tired

Fatigue is a symptom commonly associated with PD and one I experience more often each year. The term "fatigue" alone does not do justice to the experience. It is too easy to relate fatigue to being tired, overworked, or muscle aches after hard physical work. I have had these experiences in my life, and none of them compare to the fatigue I experience now with PD. In my younger years, I was an avid hiker, cyclist, a college gymnast, and coach. I was well aware of the symptoms of physical fatigue from intense exercise. But as PD progresses, I have had to redefine this different level of fatigue; thus, I use the new term **deep fatigue**.

Deep fatigue is different in its intensity and its incorporation of non-motor symptoms. Deep fatigue involves every muscle (sometimes autonomic muscle groups in my case - urinary, gastrointestinal, sexual). They are all very tired, weak, and, in my case, they are also in pain. If I have been exercising, then those muscle groups will also have a higher level of pain. In deep fatigue, it is common for me to have pain levels at 6 or 7 (level 7 is associated with spontaneous tears). I get dystonia in my legs and feet after exercise now. Sometimes, the dystonia appears even if I've not been exercising. It can wake me up in the middle of the night, lurching me out of bed, causing me to hold on to the walker and try my best to realign the foot or leg that is in severe spasm.

At the same time, my emotions have become much more intense, sometimes overwhelming, and difficult to manage. Mental energy is used to manage the pain and the emotions, leaving little energy for anything else. The duration of deep fatigue is slowly increasing for me each year. Presently, deep fatigue lasts for more than a day more often than not.

There are things which seem to make my deep fatigue

worse:

- Exercising too hard or too long
- Eating too much animal protein, or too big a meal[5]
- Not resting when needed
- Getting overheated and not drinking properly
- Being overly stressed
- Missing levodopa dose

Obviously, not doing the above is part of my rehab plan for dealing with deep fatigue. What is not so obvious is that rest and sleep are especially important.

I am an active person. I have been all my life. Taking a day to just rest is not in my nature. It feels like I am being a sloth, or the mental construct of being "lazy." Yet, I have discovered that when deep fatigue hits me, the best remedy is to do just that – take the day off! I have also found that the mind must rest with the body. Getting the mind to a quiet space is the practice of meditation, in whatever form suits the moment. At the height of deep fatigue, achieving a meditative state can be exceedingly difficult, but not impossible. There have been days when it has taken me four hours to quiet both mind and body so I can get some rejuvenating rest.

But there is a caution here to be wary of: using rest as an excuse to procrastinate. Further along in this book, I'll talk about the link of scenario looping to set-shifting issues and difficulty initiating new tasks. Basically, getting off the sofa can be problematic if I stay there too long. Perhaps this seems contradictory to my history as a highly active person, but that is the nature of the non-motor effects of PD. Once off the sofa, I make myself shift into a physical task, followed by a short rest and then some mental task. There is always some

---

[5] I found that this manifestation of fatigue related to high animal protein meals was my first indication that PD might be the cause. After enjoying a enjoy a hearty breakfast with eggs and sausage, my body would go into a state of fatigue and complete muscle collapse.

resistance to overcome – to get off the sofa – but the physical and mental rest is necessary to stopping the deep fatigue.

Terrorized by the Disease Thief

When the NYC Twin Towers fell in 2001, I was working as a crisis clinician. Although I was not at the epicenter of this disaster, its far-reaching effects were prevalent even in our rural communities. People we knew lived or worked in Manhattan. People in our communities had relatives and friends they feared were in the area of destruction. In the emergency rooms and clinical practices in our rural area, we saw an increase in the number of people needing help with anxiety-related mental health issues. The arrival of COVID-19 has produced many of the same reactions in our communities and globally. The feelings that we experience are best defined by Dr. Sheldon Solomon[6] who refers to it as *terror management* – managing the perceived threat, real or imagined, to our survival. Parkinson's disease threatens and terrorizes me, every year. It is a disease thief that invades my home, my person, my relationships, and there is nothing I can do to stop it. It will show up every year and will take something else away from me. I live with the terror.

The disease thief has ripped away three careers: professional geologist/scientist, therapist, and professor. The disease thief also took away my favorite hobbies – rock collecting, graphic arts, computer avatar gaming. These were great losses for me. These are losses of income, social network, and personal identity. A large part of how I saw myself within society was connected to these careers. I have retrained myself to use the computer as an extension of these former careers. It's not the same as face-to-face, but I'm using some of the

---

[6] Solomon, Sheldon, Greenberg, Jeff, and Pyszczynski, Tom. *The Worm at the Core: On the Role of Death in Life.* Random House, 2015.

skills I acquired over the years, and through my writing I am still teaching. Yet even as I continue to reshape my identity, I fear the disease thief lurking in the shadows waiting to invade my life again.

In my past, I actively practiced being centered and calm. I never really felt terrorized by anything, other than my military experiences in Vietnam, and those were very short-lived. I've never felt anxious about life, until recently. Stress has a way of exaggerating the emotions, and my life has been quite stressful over the last few years. We moved into a new home, we had to leave our aging pets behind, and we had trouble finding quality medical providers that could do the medical analyses necessary to see the unique form of PD that I have. There was a time it looked like it was all going to fall apart. My survival really felt like it was at risk.

I tend to feel things intensely. I can get weepy at sentimental movies and feel people's pain as if it were my own. I am a highly empathic person, and I wrote my Ph.D. dissertation on advanced levels of empathy. I have a familiarity with my own emotional states and the ability to understand others as well. But something happens with PD that changes the emotional filters, and thus changes the perception of reality connected to those emotions. It's another aspect of scenario looping breakdown.

Dealing with being terrorized by the disease thief requires terror management. These are my thoughts and actions when confronted by stress, anxiety or escalating emotional terror:

1) With intense emotion, good or bad, stop and breathe.
2) Do not act on the emotion.
3) Do not spin thoughts around the emotion.

These first three steps are important to do as early as possible in connection to the emotional experience. Waiting too long after emotion risks the potential of runaway emotion (also called limbic runaway[7]). I can spin around in my head. My body movements can tighten up at the same time. It seems like I am flailing or falling. I try to incorporate those three steps as soon as possible, followed immediately with the practice of some form of meditation. If not addressed, then the void of doing nothing will get filled up with emotional noise. After the meditation has produced a level of calm, then a rational look at the emotive events can take place.

Being terrorized by the disease thief is but one example of exaggerated emotions. There are lots of situations which can produce emotion, and with PD, exaggerated emotions. My quality of life is linked to my ability to manage my emotions. It is part of my rehab plan and includes mental attentiveness, rest, exercise, and not putting excessive or adverse chemicals or foods into my system and recognizing interpersonal or life experiences which increase the occurrence of exaggerated emotions. I confront the disease thief every day.

Human Clock Swapping – The Good, the Bad and the Ugly

I hate the bad days and what I have to say about the ugly ones is not fit for print. But the good days – well, they are delightful. I write during those times. It's not about Jekyll and Hyde mood swings – I'm talking about days where the PD symptoms present themselves as only a minor problem (the good), days when it's a struggle to get my mind and body to function well (the bad), and then days when the symptoms are most disabling (the ugly). There may be a cyclicity to the good,

---

[7] Moyer, Nancy, M.D. "Amygdala Hijack: When Emotion Takes Over," medically reviewed by Timothy J. Legg, Ph.D., CRNP, published on Healthline, April 22, 2019.

the bad and the ugly. Author John D. Palmer[8] writes about this cyclicity, saying that we are all governed by a living human clock.

Sleep is governed by the human clock, and sleep disturbances are common with the PD diagnosis. Having the strong desire to go to bed when the sun is shining, or stay awake during the dark of night, is the human clock swapping day for night. Think of a serious case of jet lag. But it is not just the sleep cycle function of the human clock that is swapped. There are many human clock cycles where the normal is swapped for the abnormal.

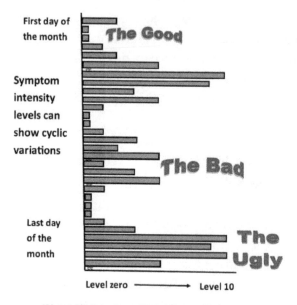

Worst PD Symptom Charted on a Scale
of 1 to 10 each day of the Month

Example Diagram* of PD Cyclic Variations
*This is an example case only! Individual variations will occur and not fit this example.

[8] Palmer, John D., M.D., Ph.D. *The Living Clock: The Orchestrator of Biological Rhythms*. Oxford University Press, 2002.

It used to be that I could get up in the morning, jump right into projects and go just about all day. My 16-hour days would be filled with accomplishments. I would have days on end where I could do this. I could excavate gem mineral specimens from deep in the earth, build stone walls, lay out perennial gardens, build paths through the woods, even build a bridge over a meandering stream. I could write and research volumes in many different domains. I loved every minute of it. This is no longer true. Those days have been swapped out for a daily cycle of times where the body and mind are available, and times where they are not – off periods.

My day has at least two off periods, with the one in the evening being the worst. Then there are bad days where the off periods are longer and more intense. In the middle of these bad days, there will be some times when it's plain ugly, when I am completely prostrate on my bed. The normal human cycle of daily life has been swapped out for this PD cycle of the good, the bad and the ugly.

Charting aspects of how the PD cycles are experienced, using a scale from 1 (least) to 10 (most), and putting that on a calendar each day, can be quite useful to learn your own personal cycles. You can chart pain, fatigue, tremors, or any other symptom that is significantly interfering with your quality of life. Charting can also help you to become more aware, and maybe even get to the point where you can say to your mate, "It feels like a bad day is right around the corner" or "Today is a level 5 day." The other piece of information which comes from charting is that you can get an idea of how long it might be until the good days return. They do return, and it helps to have some idea of when that will be when you're in the middle of the torture that accompanies the bad and the ugly days.

Communication about the good, bad, and ugly days is important for healthy relationships with family and caregivers. Using a numbering scale of 1 (least) to 10 (most) to relate symptom intensity communicates to them how the day is unfolding, so that adjustments can be made. Using this system helps family members learn to ask, "What's your level today?" Sometimes a descriptor helps to communicate "What's your pain level today?" This communication helps adjust plans for the day and helps to put in place any compensatory strategies that work during the bad days. It makes life easier on everyone.

As the disease progresses, I have found that surges of emotion affect the sensation of apathy. I identify these surges of emotion as a symptom of PD, which can be distinguished from emotions connected to significant life events.

I hate bad days and ugly ones even more, but here's the rub – exaggerated emotions are fuel for the bad days. Drop the anger and replace it with a practice of mental centering, even during the worst of it. We can't end the human clock swapping, but with a good rehab plan in place, I am learning how to balance the swap in my favor.

Taking a Careful Look at Apathy – It Could Be Motor Hesitation

Depression is often associated with PD, including apathy. But there may be a subtle difference between the two. At the risk of oversimplifying, let's define depression as a mood state of sadness and apathy as an apparent lack of motivation. Put the two together, sadness and low motivation, and the result looks like someone who has stopped enjoying life. But linking the two together may be a mistake when PD is involved because what looks like a lack of motivation may be the result of motor hesitation and difficulty with set-shifting (changing from one motor or thought activity to another). I have seen it in my own life. I feel stuck, and yet it's not due to a lack of desire but rather to an inability to move my body or my brain. It requires a careful look to see the difference.

I talk about scenario looping breakdowns in connection to freezing – a common PD motor symptom. Apathy with PD folks may be linked more to scenario looping breakdowns than to a mood disorder. With PD, it speaks to the inability to act. With a breakdown in scenario looping, it may appear the unwillingness to act is a form of freezing due to an organic neurological condition. Combine this with the "flat affect face" that can come with PD and it will appear, to the observer, that this is apathy. A careful look may reveal that sometimes it is not. It is a manifestation of scenario looping breakdowns.

Scenario looping is the brain's ability to loop through situations, exchanging and examining possible actions or responses, until the best course has been determined. This happens with language and with motor actions. In every case, the scenario determined has a starting point. If there is no external cueing from the environment to get started, we call that spontaneous initiation. An example is engaging in speech with your partner. You wouldn't always want to wait until your partner talked first (providing that external cueing). In a normal relationship, there are times where you would want to speak your mind, initiating speech spontaneously, without external cueing. Patients who have damage to areas of the brain responsible for scenario looping often will have problems with spontaneous speech. Does this mean that they are apathetic? Most likely not.

Spontaneous starting of a new motor sequence may be difficult to do for some PD patients. Another example: Mrs. Dr. C. wants me to put up a new curtain rod. This involves a series of motor tasks; getting the tools, retrieving the step stool, removing the old curtain rod, and using small screws involves many fine motor skills, which are always difficult. The curtain rod has been leaning up against the wall for a week. Is it apathy which prevents me from engaging in the task? Is it fear? It doesn't feel that way. It feels like a physical resistance to move my body in the direction of that given sequence of motor actions.

PD patients often have motor action hesitancy, and this may be misinterpreted as apathy. In the chapter "Apathy and Amotivation" by Lisa M. Shulman and Mackenzie Carpenter[9] in *Parkinson's Disease: Diagnosis and Clinical Management*, the authors identify that great care needs to be taken when ascribing the symptom of apathy to a PD patient, and that more research needs to be done.

I need to take that careful look, to be clear in my own mind that this is motor hesitancy, so that this scenario looping breakdown does not become apathy in my mind, or in the minds of those who care for me. There is that risk of mentally interpreting the motor resistance as "he doesn't care." The distinction is especially important, and I spend time in mental contemplation making the distinction clear. Muscle hesitancy, and the difficulty to initiate motor sequences, is not apathy. Understanding the difference between apathy and scenario looping breakdown is an opportunity to reframe and enlighten. Taking the time to contemplate on the difference is time well spent.

Oh, What a Drag it Is! Foot Problems as an Early Sign

Search on the Internet for early signs of Parkinson's disease. Surprisingly, you will not find foot drag on most of the lists. Yet, Ali Samil, in the chapter "Cardinal Features of Early Parkinson's Disease"[10] in *Parkinson's Disease: Diagnosis*

---

[9] Factor, Stewart A. and Weiner, William J. *Parkinson's Disease: diagnosis and clinical management*. New York: Demos Medical Publishers, 2002.
[10] Ibid.

and *Clinical Management* lists foot drag as an important early symptom. I have been dealing with the foot drag for a few years – that squeak of the sneaker on the kitchen floor when the foot catches, leaving behind a series of black scuff marks. While at a professional conference, early on in my symptoms, my foot drag caught the top edge of a stair just as I was headed to the lower level. Down I went, flailing arms and barely grasping the handrail to rescue an awful fall. But recently it has been much worse and oh, what a drag it is now.

I have had additional "up close and personal" encounters with floors and stairs and even attempting to get in the tub. It seems almost impossible that I could seriously hurt my foot walking on a flat carpeted surface, with no obstacles in the way. But that is exactly what happened. Walking barefoot on a carpet floor, my foot dragged and then my big toe jammed into the carpet – HARD! I screamed, tears flowed, and I fell to the floor weeping from the pain. The toe turned a nice purple shortly thereafter, so I'm not sure it wasn't broken, but it was most certainly badly sprained.

I don't walk barefoot anywhere now, except for a few steps in and out of the walk-in shower. Mrs. Dr. C. is constantly on the lookout for obstacles. We have removed all wall-to-wall carpeting. Instead, we have a few strategically placed braided rugs. Even these pose a significant risk. But with rug tape, they don't move. They are flat weaves and have a small rise from the floor. I know where they are and am extra cautious when traveling through those rooms.

I am surprised that there is not more mention of foot drag in the lists of early PD symptoms. If it is a cardinal early symptom, then both patients and care providers should be given the heads up (or maybe we should put our foot down) along with some guidelines on how to adjust. If a patient does have foot drag, perhaps it doesn't show up all the time, but only during off periods and deep fatigue. If the patient has a favorite pair of shoes, then perhaps signs of the foot drag can be seen on the wear pattern in the shoes. The indications of foot drag problems don't have to be as dramatic as the story I have told before foot drag becomes something that needs attention. My attention is given to the footwear I purchase, limiting my walking during deep fatigue and carefully watching my feet when changing surface levels like the curb on sidewalks – and yes, occasionally using a walking stick to navigate.

The Grouch and T.O.O.T.S. – Dealing with Irritability

When I was first diagnosed, Mrs. Dr. C. asked the neurologist, "Is there something we can do about his irritability?" The doctor responded, "I wish I had a dollar for every time a wife or caregiver made this request." It seems that this is a prevalent issue. I have talked about scenario looping breakdowns, exaggerated emotions, deep fatigue, bad days, and ugly days. All of these contribute to the occurrence of irritability, along with "off periods," which also increase irritability.

I identify myself and the emotional display of irritability as the "Grouch." The Grouch rears his growling snout and hisses at the slightest provocation or innocent question, like "what would you like for dinner?" To keep the relationship protected, T.O.O.T.S. is the necessary muzzle. T.O.O.T.S. stands for *Time Out on The Spot*. It means that you "time yourself out" – "zip the lip and take a trip." Walk away and return when calmer moods prevail.

As a therapist, and professor, I had lots of practice monitoring my internal emotive state and taking actions to prevent it from affecting others. But with PD, it became more difficult. The first time the Grouch barked back to a student in class, "putting her in her place," was something that happened on one of those bad days overlapping with high irritability. It was a shock to me that it even happened, and I went to the department chair to explain it. He just shrugged it off. I also spoke to my neurologist, saying it was like the normal filters I used to screen my emotions were not working properly. The emotions just spilled out and this Grouch took over. Now, further along with the disease, there is hardly a day that goes by when I don't have to muzzle the Grouch.

With PD irritability can be another example of exaggerated emotions. Every little thing becomes blown out of proportion. I've asked Mrs. Dr. C. not to smoke in the house and even hung a non-smoking sign (yeah – inside the house!). Yet, a cigarette still gets lit inside the house prior to walking outside. The smoke makes me nauseous and triggers the Grouch. How many little things occur in a relationship that are annoying? With the Grouch, it is not like a fly-buzzing-in-the-room type of annoying, but more like someone-elbowed-you-to-move-out-of-the-way annoying. Smelling smoke in the house after numerous reminders is sickening and close to infuriating. I put T.O.O.T.S. into action, calming down, and later I will plant a gentle reminder – again. Doing it this way prevents an argument/fight and saves the quality of the relationship. Zip the lip – save the relationship.

I find that dealing with the irritable Grouch I not only use T.O.O.T.S. but also the following:

- The 1 to 10 rating system of how bad the day is can be an approaching "Grouch" warning. I share with Mrs. Dr. C. so she knows how the day might be. For instance, "I'm at a 5 today."
- Exercise will decrease the Grouch problems.
- Deep fatigue, if not attended to, will increase Grouch problems.
- Ruminating on something annoying makes it worse – find a way to move past it.

-   I tell people what I want or need from them. If I wait for them to read my mind, I will be disappointed – and annoyed.

Stress, lack of sleep, not eating or hydrating properly, and disruptions in the daily routine can all act as triggers for the Grouch. My self-monitoring all of this as a way of keeping the Grouch muzzled is not something that happens with perfection. The Grouch still barks at Mrs. Dr. C., but the rehab plan decreases the frequency. Even more than that – the plan gives reassurance to those who love you that you are doing all that you can. Zip the lip – save the relationship.

Readers of this column published on BioNews generated many responses, with many of them wanting more information. The next two essays provide additional information, but information on being mindful and self-directing inner attention is present in many of the essays – including those that speak about conductor/exercise training.

The Itch that Must be Scratched – Impulsivity and Parkinson's

Impulsivity is a symptom commonly associated with PD, and some medications can help treat it. Impulsivity is seen as acting on urges with little thought to the consequences, that seven-year itch which feels like it must be scratched, regardless of the problems that might arise. Terror (exaggerated emotion) and irritability (the Grouch) both speak to issues centered around impulsivity.

The cognitive pathways that involve impulsivity are simplified in the graphic below with the important checkpoints labeled CP.1, CP.2 and CP.3. These checkpoints are where the impulse signals (sensory data) are heightened. The more heightened they become, the more difficult it is to alter their eventual destination of impulsive action. PD creates problems at these three checkpoints. It creates the false perception of heightened signal input, and the false impression that it is the itch that must be scratched. Recognizing this is the first step in the rehab plan.

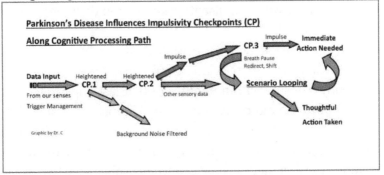

This graphic is a representation of the cognitive pathways involved and the checkpoints we can become mindful of when developing a rehabilitation plan to address impulsivity. The arrows represent the flow of data, information, into our brains (going from left to right). The first place where we can begin our impulse control practice is with trigger management. We need to identify those influences in our lives that lead us down this rocky road.

The published paper "Impulsivity and Parkinson's disease: More than just disinhibition"[11] provides an excellent discussion of the topic, as does the book chapter "Impulse Control Disorders" by Valerie Voon and Susan Fox[12]. These authors point out that PD, and the medications used to treat it, directly affect the neural pathways used to regulate

[11] Antonelli, Francesca, et al. "Impulsivity and Parkinson's disease: more than just disinhibition." *Journal of the neurological sciences* vol. 310,1-2 (2011): 202-7. doi:10.1016/j.jns.2011.06.006

[12] Factor, Stewart A., and Weiner, William, "Impulse Control Disorders," in *Parkinson's disease: diagnosis and clinical management.* New York, Demos Medical Publishing, 2007.

attention and impulse control. Any type of impulse can be affected, and those individuals with poor impulse control prior to PD onset were more likely to have more severe impulse control problems after PD onset. The contrary is also true. Those who practiced impulse control were less impacted. Rehab to deal with impulsivity requires the daily practice of impulse control.

In my introduction, I mentioned my problems with ice cream – it's a love/hate relationship. I love the taste of it and my body hates it. Within minutes of that last lingering sweet caress of sugar and chocolate, my body rebels with sneezing, cramps, and increased visits to the bathroom. Put a pint of Ben and Jerry's in the fridge, and I will devour it before the day is out. It's the itch that must be scratched. This is step two in the rehab plan to deal with impulsivity – don't put that ice cream in the fridge. Recognize the things that you just can't resist.

Step three is checkpoint awareness and adjustment. There are three checkpoints, and all three influence the perception of information coming into our brains, and thus influence impulsivity.

Checkpoint #1 is a background noise filter. Our brain doesn't consciously process everything that the senses pick up. Think of all the noises, sights, and smells that are around you every day. Normally you do not attend to them all, and do not remember them all. You simply can't process everything, so your brain filters them. I think that PD and the medications affect this filter. For me, subtle sensory stimuli have become heightened, and normal stimuli can take on an exaggerated importance. Sounds from a creaking house seem louder and more threatening; shadows seen through the corner of my eye seem like someone moving. I have been known to startle when our car is passed on the interstate by a big truck. I no longer drive, so I pay little attention to the flow of traffic around our car. But with the unexpected grinding of brakes or noisy downshifting of gears from the 18-wheelers, and my peripheral vision picking up the unanticipated appearance of a large object, the result is I'm momentarily startled.

This startle information is sent to checkpoint #2 and given emotive character – perception of danger in my immediate vicinity. In the case of the truck, it isn't going to crash into us. Mrs. Dr. C. keeps an eye on the rearview mirror while driving and knows exactly where the truck is. But I don't.

Now the fight/flight response is added to the character of the signal. The data signal has been heightened twice before getting to the last intervention checkpoint prior to becoming impulsive action. This is checkpoint #3 and it is tied to scenario looping. Step three in the rehab plan for addressing impulsivity is to focus on moderating the impact of this heightened signal input. This can be done through various brain-training practices, including the three steps I mentioned above: awareness, trigger management, checkpoint control.

Train the Brain to Stop the Train – Moderating Impulsivity with PD

Brain training happens all the time, but in PD rehabilitation, we want to put in place training which will limit the effects of the disease. To train the brain, it is important to be mindful of what the brain is doing, to put in place a constant practice of mental attentiveness. This is a specific type of mindfulness aimed at compensating for issues connected to PD. The rehab plan is aimed at putting a skilled conductor inside your brain who is trained to slow down and eventually stop the impulsivity train.

	Triggers	**Checkpoint 1**
Mental Attention	Pay attention to all the people, places and things that are triggers for the impulsive action.	Heightened Startle Understand that the sensory input can be heightened and create an abnormal startle response. Become aware of when this is happening.
Slowing it Down	Slow down thought and action enough to become aware of when the triggers are present.	Don't react to the startle response. Slow it down.
Changing the Course	Take steps to either remove the triggers, or **yourself** from the triggers, without doing harm.	Use T.O.O.T.S.

	Checkpoint 2	Checkpoint 3
Mental Attention	Heightened Emotion Understand that exaggerated emotion does happen. Pay attention to when it happens. Learn about the connection to both trigger and startle response.	Thought Enhanced Heightened input demands the attention of your brain, but when the input is distorted, then the attention can be also. Become aware of how this happens.
Slowing it Down	Don't react to the exaggerated emotion. Slow it down.	Slow the mind down when input is exaggerated. Be on the **lookout** for spinning around on an emotion or turning a startle response into a "real" perception.
Changing the Course	Use T.O.O.T.S.	Use scenario looping training and meditation to place your mind in a more health promoting place.

The general application of Mindfulness as MBSR (Mindfulness Based Stress Reduction) has yet to provide clear scientific evidence for its efficacy in treating Parkinson's patients.[13] The problem is that the studies are sometimes poorly designed. This is not the same as saying mindfulness is not helpful. Mindfulness, when practiced frequently, may result in changing the brain structure in PD patients.[14] I am a strong believer that mindfulness is a valid and constructive way of handling many of my reactions and management of symptoms. I'll return to this theme in several essays.

For now, I think this is the way that we train the brain to stop the train of impulsivity – we act, and think, in a new way so that the structure of the brain is changed. The brain is made to be plastic, to change in response to what we do with it.

When properly applied to PD and impulsivity, mindfulness is composed of three parts: 1) mental attentiveness (focusing attention where it is needed); 2) slowing down the impulse; and 3) changing the course. When putting the rehabilitation plan in place, mindfulness uses these three components, directed at the triggers of impulsivity and the three checkpoints. The table above explains the application of mindfulness to impulsivity.

The key to impulsivity management is to eventually turn the training into habit, into almost automatic responses to those heightened responses that happen at each checkpoint. This is how we train the brain to stop the train of impulsivity – or at least slow it down.

---

[13] McLean, Gary, et al. "Mindfulness-based stress reduction in Parkinson's disease: a systematic review." *BMC Neurology* (2017) 17:92 DOI 10.1186/s12883-017-0876-4

[14] Pickut, Barbara A., et al. "Mindfulness based intervention in Parkinson's disease leads to structural brain changes on MRI: A randomized controlled longitudinal trial." *Clinical Neurology and Neurosurgery*, Volume 115, Issue 12, 2013, Pages 2419-2425.

Computer Gaming as Therapy for Parkinson's Disease[15]

The brain is a plastic organ and it continually reshapes itself in response to the stimuli it receives and how that stimuli is processed. That old saying "use it or lose it" applies even in the face of a challenging disease like Parkinson's. Computer gaming can help with brain training, exercising the brain to slow the progression of the disease.

Recent research on video gaming and treatment for PD shows it can help with physical issues such as gait and balance.[16] There is a certain amount of brain, eye, and hand coordination in video gaming. The key to successful use of computer gaming is to find the right match of game to person and level of difficulty. The game must be challenging, but not too much to be discouraging for a new player. It also must be rewarding and enjoyable (there is that dopamine factor to consider). There is a "sweet spot" in gaming where, like Goldilocks, you find just the right fit. I find this in games where I can play it at various levels. Not only can you find a comfortable level for your own style of playing, but you can also change the level depending on whether it is a good day or a bad day with Parkinson's.

I look for video games that offer exercise for geographical memory, eye-hand coordination, speech, and problem solving

---

[15] This essay published on Parkinson's News Today resulted in Dr. C. being interviewed by *Thrive* newsletter for Parkinson's patients in their January 2021 "Gamification Issue". The reader can subscribe at home.thrivenewsletter.com for free newsletters about Parkinson's disease topics.

[16] Computer Games Help People with Parkinson's Disease. A pilot study by UCSF School of Nursing and Red Hill Studios. Small Business Innovative Research grants totaling $1.1 million from the *National Institute of Neurological Disorders and Stroke* – part of the National Institutes of Health. Published online 2020.

(scenario looping) at a variety of levels. It is also a place for the Grouch to go when T.O.O.T.S. needs to be applied and where impulsivity can be applied with fewer consequences than in the real world. Have the urge to buy? Then earn virtual money and buy virtual things. Have some frustration? Then enter the video game world and work it out on some monsters. Controlling my pain is a difficult problem for me. Spending time in the virtual world can help. Want a sense of accomplishment? Help build a community while also making yourself a strong avatar. It is a place where you can find that "sweet spot" while contributing to building a support community.

It may seem counterintuitive to say that fighting monsters or building a virtual community is relaxing, but that is what I experience. Conversations I have had with others indicate that this is a common experience. I often have clarity of mind while playing, and some of my ideas for writing pop up in the middle of the game. There is the added benefit of meeting new challenges. Keeping the brain in shape is one way to help stave off dementia and the effects of aging. I enjoy problem-solving, so the games that offer that to me are much more enjoyable. In a goal-driven game, I find that new and novel situations challenge my thinking. There is the dopamine effect that happens when I'm successful within a game that offers many ways to experience success. Can't get much better than this – having good clean fun and slowing down the progression of PD!

One more note – I do use adaptive equipment to help me play the game. I have a large track ball on my dominant hand and a keypad with a thumb joystick on my other hand. It takes a little while to learn how to use this equipment, but the reward is a greater success rate inside the virtual world. I also have a headset with a microphone. There is plenty of opportunity to speak with others within the community of players. However, addiction to gaming can be a problem, and too much time gaming can have negative consequences. One can enjoy the challenge, but be aware of any potential impulsivity issues you may be facing.

The Pacman Cometh – Parkinson's Disease Gobbles up Time

It used to be that I could put long hours into just about anything I tackled – research, counseling, painting, writing, and gardening. But PD gobbles up time, like the video game Pacman gobbling up dots as it chases the ghosts. Even though I am retired, there is less free time to use to accomplish personal goals because every day the Parkinson's-Pacman cometh.

Here is a list of the ways the PD-Pacman gobbles up my time:

- Bad days and "off periods" require a commitment of time to manage.
- Medical appointments and travel to them.
- Pain and fatigue, and more rest needed to help manage them.
- Any illness, like the flu or colds, is more intense and takes more time get well.
- Heightened emotions along with stress of any kind, good or bad, requires more time to manage.
- The overall rehabilitation plan to address all the issues associated with PD, which I have mentioned in past essays, takes quite a bit of time.

Many evenings, as I get to the end of the day, it feels like nothing was accomplished. It's a plaguing voice and annoying – and not just to me. Mrs. Dr. C. has heard it so many times that she is now responding, "I'm going to have that on your tombstone – 'Here lies Dr. C. He died wishing he got more done in his life.'"

There are tons of magazine articles and books on time management. But PD has its own special problems that need to be considered when seeking to apply time management strategies. Think of time like money – you only have so much you can spend each month. You can't get back what the PD-Pacman gobbles up, although you can decrease what the Pacman consumes by implementing a personally tailored rehabilitation plan. After that, it is important to cherish the time that is available and to allocate it in a meaningful and constructive fashion.

Misdirected attention is the Pacman of PD. It consumes time in two ways. First, by getting us to get off task; second, due to the set-shifting problems connected to scenario looping, we can end up staying off task. It may even feel quite difficult to get back on track. After physical exercise and good medical care, mental attentiveness is the third most important treatment focal point for early PD folks. Like physical exercise, mental attentiveness needs to be practiced daily, which is one of the reasons for my recommending virtual reality game playing.

Capitalize on using the good days, and the good hours in a day, when they occur. Without being fierce about it, jump into those good days and focus on accomplishing tasks which have rich meaning and purpose. There are times during the illness where the mind is more lucid. Use those times wisely with directed attention. Be patient and allow those times to arrive. Be flexible on the mild days. Get done what you can and then be willing to rest. On the bad days, and especially the ugly days, be willing to let it go. As boring as it seems, rest is needed to limit the extent of the bad days.

With these suggestions in place, make a schedule. Make broad goals and then weekly goals. Use those good times during the week to apply yourself, with mental attentiveness, to those goals. This is a little bit different than saying, "On

Monday I will do this, and Tuesday, that." Instead, it is a flexible schedule which says, "I would like to get this done by the end of the week." Then, when the good times, the lucid times, arrive, you get that weekly goal done.

Finally – keeping track of appointments on a calendar (on paper, computer, and cell phone) is important. I find that sometimes I just can't get to an appointment. The drive is too much to endure, my body is rebelling, or the weather is bad. Lately, the precautions for the pandemic are impacting provider availability and my willingness to expose myself in a large medical institution. For those of you who can access telehealth, I encourage that. Keeping providers up to date on your physical and mental status cannot be overstated.

A New Year's Resolution: Quiet Down the Old Tapes

In the previous essay on time management, I mentioned a nagging inner voice saying, "You did not get enough done today." This is tied to an old tape, inner dialog left by the voices of parents and childhood teachers, that said, "You are never going to amount to anything." The inner drive to continually produce is an effort on my part to quiet down this old tape. But with PD, and getting older, the cost of this nagging inner dialog has become too much. An interesting management technique is proposed by author Kara Brown to suppress these memories: "To learn more about how to stop past thoughts, researchers looked at three modes of eliminating memories. They found that while replacing thoughts and clearing the mind removes memories quickly, suppressing memories is better at thoroughly removing them."[17]

The inner drive to always be doing something, to produce something, is also tied to a sense of identity. The holiday times are filled with meeting friends and family where the conversation often inquires, "What have you been doing?" "Doing" is connected to how we describe ourselves to others and our self-identity. But, as mentioned in the time management essay, PD consumes the time that could be used for doing those things that are connected to self-identity. The sense of self begins to shift, and the old tapes, once silenced by a healthy productive life, are now emboldened by the disease.

Everyone has old tapes tied to memories, some more intense than others. My New Year's resolutions usually focus on the most annoying one for me. Perhaps it has become that way because PD makes it harder to find the self I once knew when I did not grapple with the disease. Since I can't find, feel, know, or sense that old self in the same way, there is an emptiness. Part of how I knew myself seems absent, and that emptiness gets filled with the noise from the old tapes. I can't use "doing" as a functional way to address this anymore, so it is my New Year's resolution to find a better way.

The search for self amid PD is a winding path through the forest of symptoms and steps taken to embrace a high quality of life. It is a forest path filled with obstacles, and it can become one's negative self-identity. But there is difference between saying, "There stands that Parkinson's guy" and saying, "There stands Dr. C. – he has Parkinson's." It may seem like a subtle difference, but it is important because linking one's self-identity too closely with the disease also creates a link to negative self-dialog, like "You are a diseased person." This then raises the volume of the old tape.

---

[17] "I'm a Neuroscientist, and This Is How to Stop Past Thoughts from Lingering," by Kara J. Brown, published on Well+Good Healthy Mind, January 4, 20

The disease should never become our self-identity, but given how much time is spent and how much conversation is shared focusing on the disease, it is difficult to not become the disease. The cognitive aspects of PD make it harder to stay in touch with that healthy self-identity. Who am I? How do others view me now that I have this disease? Answers to these questions help me to keep in touch with a self-identity I have developed and strengthened over five decades. Even though I am trying to replace negative internal dialog with positive internal dialog as a regular practice, it just seems a bit harder these days. So, my New Year's resolutions are sent to me, Dr. C., struggling to sit with a healthy sense of self. It is a resolution wish sent along with gentleness. It is sent with hope, kindness, and an infinite well of patience.

Looking for Lightness of Being – Meditation and Parkinson's Disease

Living with PD is a daily battle with the loss of both motor and cognitive functions. Effort must be put into a plan of action that reduces the impact of the disease – a rehabilitation plan. This effort is daily, sometimes hourly, and it can be exhausting. Living with PD is like carrying a large backpack of rocks. It is at times a crushing burden and overwhelming. Sometimes I can carry it – other times the pack shifts and slips, throwing off my mental and emotional balance. There needs to be balance in my life so that the work I do on my rehab plan does not consume me. I must spend time looking for lightness of being to balance out the heavy PD burden. This can be done through a regular practice of meditation.

There are many ways to practice meditation: sit and listen to calming music, sit and gaze at a fireplace, practice Tai Chi, or exercise with rhythmic breathing. These are all aimed at relieving stress, easing the burdens of life, and entering the quiet mind. It is within the quiet mind that lightness of being can be experienced to calm the noise in both body and mind. There are books providing instructions on how to do this, but few deal directly with implementing them for PD.

Practicing meditation with PD presents some unique challenges. The meditation practice starts with calming the body, and this is the first obstacle that PD makes more difficult.

Repetitive motor activities like cycling, Tai Chi, or gardening are helpful when combined with focused breathwork. Focused breathwork is diaphragmatic breathing where you focus your full attention on the breathing. Guided meditation, either from a teacher, in person, or a recording, can help with this process of shifting attention. This shifting of attention is the second obstacle PD makes more difficult.

Once past the first two obstacles, you should feel a little more relaxed and sense the door to the quiet mind opening. But I am prevented from getting to that door by a third obstacle.

This third obstacle is heightened emotions and difficulty in regulating them. I have written about how PD heightens the impulse signals to the brain. During the meditation process, the signal-to-noise ratio changes, meaning as one practice quieting the mind, the internal noise goes down and the signals connected to emotion appear louder. Sometimes very loud! The quiet mind is a mental state where the noise of the world, the body and the self are silenced, while at the same time maintaining a sense of peace and safety. It is something I practiced for decades and then lost touch with over these years while in battle with PD and all its consequences. Now, as my life has become more stable, I am returning to the practice and finding it much more difficult. I feel like a novice struggling with all the obstacles I used to walk around with ease. This third obstacle does impede my success with meditation and looking for lightness of being.

As I once helped patients to find a place of peace and safety, together we would often experience loud emotions. These are emotions connected to things we feel need to be given attention, consciously or subconsciously. They are like boulders in the path, obstacles blocking the way forward to the quiet mind. But one can learn to walk around them. As I write this, I am reminded of this and the tender patience I should offer to myself.

Once past the boulders of emotion, you then arrive at the doorstep of the quiet mind. Looking for lightness of being requires opening that door and exploring the rooms beyond. I have memories of doing this. They point out familiar landmarks for me. PD has made looking for lightness of being much more difficult for me, but not impossible. I have felt glimpses of peace, and deep calmness. Looking for lightness of being ties into my New Year's resolution. For me to quiet down the old tapes (which are my emotional boulders in the path), I need to have a new mental state to go to. I can't just remove the tapes and leave a void, because that void will be quickly filled back in with the old mental habits. Looking for lightness of being will be a lifetime adventure.

Bananas and Beans, not Burgers: High Protein Meals and Levodopa

No one told me breakfast bacon, ham, or sausage would make me feel awful! I had seen my off periods worsen after a heavy meat meal, but I shrugged it off as "just a bad off period." Now, after being on the medication for many years, I am positive that animal protein meals are a serious issue. Overlapping a high-meat meal with the levodopa can result in not just an off period, but an entire day that feels like an off period. "Bananas and beans, not burgers" is the mantra to remind me that diet is particularly important in the development of a rehab plan for folks with PD.

I am not a nutritionist. I am writing from the perspective of a PD patient warrior and rehab clinician. But there is more research recognizing and suggesting how changes to your diet will help alleviate some symptoms of your PD.

The American Parkinson's Disease Association (APDA) recognizes that levodopa crosses the wall of the small intestine via molecules in the intestinal wall that transport amino acids. When dietary protein (beef, chicken, pork, fish, eggs, nuts, and dairy) is also present in the small intestine, then there are fewer transporters available for levodopa to use. We may experience the "protein effect" when the medication competes with a high-protein meal. One of the most compelling statements in a 2014 study published in *Frontiers in Aging Neuroscience* is that in Parkinson's disease, "[A] growing body of evidence suggests that nutrition may play an important role."[18]

Nyholm and Lennernas reported on "irregular gastrointestinal drug absorption in Parkinson's disease"[19]. They state that levodopa transit time in the small intestine is approximately three hours. Therefore, gastric emptying is a major determining factor for onset of symptom relief. It is the time it takes for food to empty from the stomach and enter the small intestine. When gastric emptying is delayed in PD, it has the potential to cause motor fluctuations, known to us as off periods. "In PD patients, gastroparesis has the potential to affect nutrition and quality of life, as well as the absorption of

[18] Seidl, Stacey E., et al. "The emerging role of nutrition in Parkinson's disease." *Frontiers in Aging Neuroscience*, 6 (2014):36.

[19] Nyholm, Dag and Hans Lennernas in Expert Opinion on *Drug Metabolism Toxicology*, 4:2, 193-203, DOI: 101517/17425255.4.s.193. 2008

PD medications, including L-dopa. This reduced absorption of L-dopa has implications for the control of the PD motor symptoms for which it is administered.[20] The researchers state, "Based on this review, we conclude that while gastric emptying has been reported to be frequently delayed in PD, the existing data do not permit definitive conclusions concerning its true prevalence, relationship to the underlying disease process, relevance to PD management, or the optimal therapy of related GI symptoms. Further study of these important issues is, therefore, required."[21]

Another study at the University of Washington's Department of Environmental and Occupational Health Sciences in Seattle reported the possible association between Parkinson's disease and eating vegetables containing small amounts of dietary nicotine. Peppers, tomatoes, potatoes, and eggplants had protective potential, especially if study subjects had never smoked, or smoked less than 10 years. Dr. Michael Greger writes in Nutrition Facts[22] that ingested dietary nicotine may be significant and explains: "[The researchers] ... found none in eggplant, only a little in potatoes, some in tomatoes, but the most in bell peppers. The researchers found that more peppers meant more protection. And, as we might expect, the effects of eating nicotine-containing foods were mainly evident in nonsmokers, as the nicotine from smoke would presumably blot out any dietary effect."

There's also research that there is a relationship between

[20] Heetun, Z.S, and Quigley, E.M. "Gastroparesis and Parkinson's disease: a systematic review." *Parkinsonism & Related Disorders.* 2012 Jun;18(5):433-40. doi: 10.1016/j.parkreldis.2011.12.004. Epub 2011 Dec 29. PMID: 22209346.

[21] Ibid.

[22] "Treating Parkinson's Disease With Diet" by Michael Greger, M.D., FACLM. Published on Nutritionfacts.org on August 29, 2013.

your microbiome[23] (the microorganisms in your body), Parkinson's disease, and improved gut health. Work by Dr. George Tetz and his colleagues (*Scientific Reports,* July 2018) examined the viruses that live in your gut, as well as the role the microbiome may play in Parkinson's. According to Parkinson.org, the study "has sparked the idea that we might be able to improve the symptoms if we change the microbiome through diet or other ways... These bacteria play a role in the processes that produce dopamine and affect the intestine's ability to absorb."[24] *The China Study* by Campbell and Campbell[25] is an example of solid research on diet and illustrates the negative impact of a heavy meat diet.

Like many aspects of Parkinson's symptoms, the protein effect is highly variable. Some people do not experience it at all. Others are extremely sensitive to protein's effect on medication absorption. This concern was presented at my local PD support group and the group PD warriors and caregivers agreed almost unanimously with experiencing adverse effects.

It typically becomes more of an issue as PD progresses.

---

[23] "Go with your Gut" by Mercola, J. published on Mercola.com, January 2013.

[24] "What's Hot in PD? The Not So Hidden Viruses in the Parkinson Disease Microbiome" by Michael S. Okun, MD. Published on Parkinson.org/blog on October 5, 2018. *See also* "Bacteriophages, the Microbiome, and Parkinson Disease: Possible Treatment Implications." Journal Watch Neurology, 2018.

[25] Campbell, T. Colin. *The China Study.* T. Colin Campbell, Ph.D. of Cornell University, in partnership with researchers at Oxford University and the Chinese Academy of Preventive Medicine. The data was published in the following monograph: Chen, J., Campbell, T.C., Li, J., Peto, R. "A Study of the Characteristics of 65 Chinese Counties." *Diet, Lifestyle and Mortality in China.* A joint publication of: Oxford University Press, Cornell University Press, and The People's Medical Publishing House, 1990.

The APDA[26] suggests that if a person discovers they experience the protein effect, there are two potential strategies to try. One is to refrain from eating protein during the day and instead, eat protein at night when medication effect is less critical. The second is to distribute protein intake evenly throughout the day so that medication absorption is enhanced in that time.

The solution I have found works best for me includes two parts. First, I space the levodopa dosing so that it occurs between meals to minimize the absorption issues. Second, I eat the moderate meat meal of the day for lunch, with limited amounts at dinner and breakfast. I seem to do fairly well with an egg at breakfast or small portions of chicken or fish in the evening. As the China Study and other researchers have revealed, decreasing meat intake is a good change for all of us. Bananas and beans, not burgers.

Finding Words to Describe Parkinson's Pain

The pain which can accompany PD is unique, and finding words to describe the experience is difficult. Not all those with the PD diagnosis experience pain. But there are some PD patients, like me, for which pain is the major symptom and quite disabling. It is important to find the words to describe the pain experience as clearly as possible. There is no "grin and bear it" nor is this "a pity party." Instead, this is a search for accurate articulation of the pain experience to maintain quality of life.

Pain has been associated with Parkinson's, but many providers often do not recognize the correlation, especially if the patient is in the early stages of the disease. However, a

---

[26] "What we know about avoiding particular foods & supplements for Parkinson's" by Dr. Rebecca Gilbert. Published on American Parkinson's Disease Association website April 22, 2019.

recent study, "Pain: A marker of prodromal Parkinson's disease?" was presented at the recent 2018 World Congress on Parkinson's Disease and Related Disorders (IAPRD)[27], held in Lyon, France. This was reported in Parkinson's News Today.[28] The problem can be compounded by the PD pain that resembles pain from other disease processes, especially as the patient ages and faces a multitude of other conditions such as arthritis, spine degeneration, poor muscle conditioning, and so on.

The American Parkinson Disease Association published research[29] that supports the identification of pain with Parkinson's. They also highlight if the pain is relieved with dopaminergic medication during a pattern of painful sensation that correlates to "off" episodes, more credence can be given to the fact that the pain is PD-related.

Pain has lots of sources, particularly as we age. In my case, pain with PD can be distinguished by the following:

1) The progression of body pain seems related to the progression of the disease.
2) Levodopa works to reduce the pain.
3) The pain is worse during off periods.

There is also a particular character to the PD pain that I experience. The best ways to describe this character is stinging, sometimes needle jabbing, irritating tingling,

---

[27] Acharya M.K., Das S. , Ganguly G., Das S.K. "Pain: A marker of prodromal Parkinson's disease?" Bangur Institute of Neurosciences, Neurology, Kolkata, India, 2 IPGMER, Kolkata, India, 3 Bangur Institute of Neurosciences, Kolkata, India. Abstract published in the proceedings of the *World Congress on Parkinson's Disease and Related Disorder: A Comprehensive education program*. August 19-22, 2018. Available at International Association of Parkinsonism and Related Disorders.

[28] "Pain May Be Early Detector of Parkinson's, Study Suggests" by Jose Marques Lopes, Ph.D. Published on Parkinson's News Today, August 27, 2018.

[29] "Is Pain a Symptom of Parkinson's Disease?" by Dr. Rebecca Gilbert. Published on APDAparkinson.org, August 27, 2019.

burning, and a muscle heaviness with increased pain on movement. This can occur over large regions of the body and varies in severity. At the worst of times, it can reach level 7, inducing spontaneous tears, and last several days. Finding words to describe when this PD pain happens is an important part of quality care.

PD with episodic chronic pain is disabling in several ways. First, high levels of pain interfere with clear thinking. Second, high levels of pain induce the "fight or flight" response, and this interferes with emotion management. Third, the amount of energy it takes to manage this is very tiring, even more so in the face of the deep fatigue associated with PD. There is much more to PD chronic pain that just the body symptoms. PD pain is a total experience that touches thoughts, feelings, and relationships. Finding the words – even if it is a struggle – to describe your pain experience is an important part of maintaining quality of life in the face of a difficult diagnosis.

Over the years of having the PD diagnosis, I have watched the progression. I have taken the warrior stance to do all I can to slow down the progression. My toughest battle is with the total experience of PD chronic pain. Large blocks of time disappear into the fog of war. Over time, I learned the importance of communicating about the pain daily, sometimes multiple times a day. Mrs. Dr. C. asks, "Where are you today?" I will say, "I'm at level 5" followed by a quick mention of the most bothersome symptoms. In the past, I have kept track of the pain levels over the span of several months. This is all part of finding the words to describe the PD pain experience.

I have been a "communicator" most of my life. But it's still a struggle finding words to describe the unique character of the PD pain experience.

Note: This column received more comments than any other column out of the 100 published on *Parkinson's News Today* between 2018 and 2020. The comments reflect the diversity of the PD experience. There are several essays in this book that address chronic pain.

The C.H.R.O.N.D.I. Creed – A Parkinson's Disease Warrior's Guide

The challenges of any chronic disease require the mental attitude of a warrior. Like the code of the Samurai, the CHRONDI Creed is both a guide for battle and for living. CHRONDI is an acronym made from the first letters in the words "chronic disease." They stand for each part of the Creed as follows:

C – compassion
H – happiness
R – rehabilitation
O – others
N – nature
D – death
I – individuality

Below is the CHRONDI Creed in its self-affirming dialog that I use with each statement in this chronic disease warrior's Creed.

C – Compassion: I will act compassionately toward others and find gentleness toward self.

H – Happiness: I will seek the inner bliss of happiness that is not material in nature.

R – Rehabilitation: I will apply courage and mindfulness to my part in fighting the disease.

O – Others: I will genuinely communicate to others my experiences and maintain an attitude of gratitude for their help.

N – Nature: I will take time to embrace nature and all its beauty.

<u>D - Death</u>: I will find the courage to face the terror of "death" and not let it control me.

<u>I - Individuality</u>: I will continue to express my individuality, purpose, beyond the disease.

These CHRONDI Creed statements are short "I" statement that can not only be self-affirming, but they also change how a disease affects one's life. If these statements become an inner dialog, a way of thinking and acting, then they can contribute to quality of life.

Compassion, as a way of thinking and acting, is the foundation of the CHRONDI Creed. It is a state of being that is expressed both externally and internally. In the face of a chronic disease, this is certainly difficult. But it doesn't have to be perfect saintly compassion. It can start with small steps – just taking the time each day to do something for another. In addition, this sense of a gentle kindness can be a kind word to self: "You did well today."

Happiness is not tied to the material things, although it may appear to be. Denzel Washington is attributed with the quote, "You'll never see a U-Haul behind a hearse. ... Now, I've been blessed to make hundreds of millions of dollars in my life. I can't take it with me, and neither can you. It's not how much you have but what you do with what you have." Happiness is tied to an internal state of being often connected to events, not possessions. We are happy because we feel happy. There is a state of bliss that can accompany times when an event generates an ecstasy, a bliss of happiness. Happiness is an important part of well-being in the face of chronic disease. Returning to the bliss can be as simple as finding joy and laughter.

Rehabilitation means that we will do our part in supporting all treatment modalities that are used to fight the chronic disease. We can continue to educate ourselves – and sometimes our providers – of successful treatment or failed treatment. Not everything we try is going to work. It may be that one "solution" is good for some and not for others. The main objective is to keep trying. Research information. Don't make assumptions that everything is known about Parkinson's disease and nothing new is being researched. There is so much we know we don't know.

Others stands for all relationships in our lives. The statement is a promise to speak in an authentic manner with a sense of gratitude. With PD, social connections change. We may no longer be able to participate in activities we shared with others because the physical challenges cannot be surmounted. Relationships change because the wife or husband becomes a caretaker, assuming new roles in daily lives. Children may be reluctant to face the idea that a parent is now more dependent on them. A relationship dynamic is changed and many, not only the person with PD, must adapt.

Nature, and all its beauty, when incorporated into life, can make a difference in our well-being. A stroll through the woods, or a park, while maintaining a quiet mind, can add to our quality of life. Gardening is also therapeutic. I write more about this in other essays in this book. It is a mainstay of my personal rehab plan.

"Death" has quotes around it because it refers to those things the disease has taken and will continue to take with a brutal finality. There is "terror" in facing this "death." Terror management takes courage and a practice of finding a calm center in the middle of the storm. Expressing individuality is balanced against the time used by the chronic disease, the thought and emotion that the chronic disease consumes. Find your inner voice, your unique identity, and your purpose. Let that light which is you continue to shine forth.

The CHRONDI Creed is a list of statements I use to help me as a warrior against the ever-worsening effects of Parkinson's disease. Not for a single day can I achieve a level of perfection with all aspects of the creed. Perfection is an illusion, perhaps a nightmare. Rather, I hold these statements as an inner dialog, as a path to follow, as a gentle guide for living. It is in this way that the CHRONDI Creed improves my quality of life.

The Compassionate Warrior in the Battle Against PD

The C in the CHRONDI Creed,[30] a warrior's guide in the battle against PD, is for **compassion**. It may seem odd labeling a warrior as compassionate. Normally we picture the warrior as fierce, brave, courageous, and strong. Compassion is not often associated with such an image. But, in the battle against a chronic disease, being both a warrior and compassionate has important benefits. The compassionate warrior brings a special set of armor and weapons to the battle against a chronic disease.

Compassion is the mindset upon which the strength and courage of the warrior is set in motion. In my research, I have defined compassion[31] as empathy plus wisdom: Empathy being defined as the ability to sense and hear the suffering of others, and wisdom being the ability to do something to reduce that suffering. Compassion is about the reduction of suffering in the world around you.

The first step to becoming a compassionate warrior is making a commitment to a life of compassion, a philosophy of compassion.[32] The second step is to realize that you can change your behavior so that you contribute less to the

---

[30]The CHRONDI Creed: A Guide for Parkinson's Warriors. Dr. C. "Possibilities with Parkinson's." Published on Parkinson's News Today, February 8, 2019.

[31] "Seeking the Soul of Life: A quest of compassion and finding our 'true self' in the midst of a hectic world" by Dr. C. at www.DrC.life

[32] "The Compassionate Journey" by Dr. C. at www.DrC.life

suffering of those around you.

The third step is realizing that you can act in a way that helps reduce the suffering of those around you, and without sacrificing your own well-being. In fact, this path of the compassionate warrior promotes personal well-being.

The challenges of living with PD are many. The most obvious are the motor and coordination issues that impact every movement. But there are emotion issues that are equally impactful: Impulse control issues, grief/loss and depression, anxiety, and anger. Add to this what many Parkinson's patients find as a decreased ability to manage these emotions. When the actions connected to these emotions spill out into life, the consequences can be costly and add to an already arduous chronic disease battle. This is where the practice of compassion plays an important role. Practicing compassion is very much a scenario looping skill[33] and, as such, is good brain training for people with PD. Without doing so directly, the practice of compassion helps us to moderate those emotions and decrease the consequences they can have in life.

It may seem odd saying that acting in a compassionate manner has benefits to one's self. It is not the goal of compassion, nor is it in the mindset of compassion. It is simply a positive side effect. Compassion has its focus on the other person. The skill with which a person can do this depends upon their history with practicing compassion, but you don't have to be an expert to have it make a difference. Practicing compassion at any level is good for relationships, and healthy relationships improve the quality of life for anyone with a chronic disease. The compassionate mindset is also one of gentleness, which can be (should be) applied to self in healthy doses. Being a compassionate warrior does not mean we

---

[33] "A New Look at Freezing: 'Scenario Looping Breakdowns' as an Early Symptom." Dr. C. "Possibilities with Parkinson's," Published on Parkinson's News Today, September 28, 2018.

sacrifice our own well-being for the sake of another. Two persons in the rowboat, each manning the oars, makes the journey easier.

After practicing compassion for some time, one can move from contemplated action, to the first action taken, to the first thought considered, and then to living as a compassionate warrior. I have been training as a compassionate warrior for decades, and PD has set me back. But as a compassionate warrior, I continue to work at this, as hard as any warrior would who is preparing for battle. The compassionate warrior does this preparation along with meditation and a calm mind.[34] It is a commitment to living and it serves as a foundation for the other parts of the CHRONDI Creed. In addition, the other parts of the CHRONDI Creed help to support this foundation, to make it easier to become a compassionate warrior against the chronic disease of Parkinson's.

Holding on to Happiness – But Not too Tightly

Life, liberty, and the pursuit of happiness – the H in the CHRONDI Creed refers to happiness. Happiness can be an elusive thing when battling with a chronic disease like Parkinson's. There are so many things that get in the way of experiencing happiness: pain, deep fatigue, irritability, the time and grief accompanying the losses. Trying to hold on to even small moments of happiness is a challenge. It is possible to experience moments of happiness in the face of a chronic disease if one holds the moment gently – not too tightly.

Happiness is a state of mind and includes a broad range of

---

[34] "Meditation and Parkinson's Disease: Looking for Lightness of Being." Dr. C. "Possibilities with Parkinson's," Published on Parkinson's News Today, January 11, 2019.

phenomena, e.g., gratitude, inspiration, beauty, awe, laughter, compassion, deep calmness/peace, joy, love, exhilaration, ecstasy, and bliss. The experience of happiness can have a connection to just one, or several, of these phenomena. Let's take a mental excursion together. Visualize in your mind the last time you were happy and try to feel how you felt at that time.

Were any of the above phenomena part of your memory? Remembering happiness is helpful in reminding us what it felt like, of what the experience may look like again. It can help us to see it in the smallest of moments throughout our lives. It is not a practice of grasping after happiness. Happiness is like a butterfly flitting from flower to flower. We take in the beauty and the rich sensual experience and hold it gently in our minds. If we were to grasp the butterfly, we would destroy the experience.

Gently holding happiness, without grasping, is tied to a compassionate way of being. So much of our unhappiness is tied to grasping, to misperceptions, and to poor communication in relationships. The practice of compassion is about experiencing the needs of others and then moving beyond to a place of well-being. It is a shift out of suffering. Walking the path of the compassionate warrior is filled with happiness experiences accompanied by the knowledge of shifting perception. Scrooge, in Charles Dickens' *A Christmas Carol*, wasn't happy until he experienced a shift in perception and discovered his compassionate feelings.

I don't expect myself to experience happiness all the time. It is just too unrealistic for where I am in my personal development as a compassionate warrior battling a chronic disease. I seek small moments each day, not by grasping for them but by looking for them, like looking at the butterfly, and then gently holding the moment in my mind. Then I am grateful for that moment and not sad when it naturally fades into the next experience as part of the day. This feeling of happiness is not induced by drugs or alcohol, which bring artificial happiness. It is a happiness that comes from the practice of allowing the mind to experience the small – and big – moments of happiness that occur. I do my best to begin and end each day with a confirmation (mantra, prayer) of specific gratitude, meaning it is not a statement of general gratitude, but one aimed at something specific in my life. It is a way of holding the door open for those happiness moments.

Perhaps, happiness brain training can be helpful for those suffering from PD because of the link to dopamine production. I haven't seen any credible scientific research on this, but speaking personally, I find the practice to be quite helpful.

Rehabilitation is About A Path to Well-Being

Rehabilitation, the R in the CHRONDI Creed,[35] is about the path to well-being. It is a path that all who battle with a chronic disease, like Parkinson's, seek to walk every day. A well-designed rehab plan can make that journey easier. Think of a rehab plan as an expanded treatment plan that includes all aspects of living the good life. This essay will look at the key features of a successful rehab plan for use in the battle against chronic disease.

My Ph.D. is in rehabilitation counseling with many years of writing clinical rehab plans for patients with brain injuries. Most often, a rehab plan is thought of as a "back to work" plan following an injury. But it can also be thought of as a "back to well-being" plan when facing a chronic disease. A rehab plan includes medical care, but also everything else that helps to promote well-being. It is a total well-being plan that includes

---

[35] "A New Look at Freezing: 'Scenario Looping Breakdowns' as an Early Symptom." Dr. C. "Possibilities with Parkinson's," Published on Parkinson's News Today, September 28, 2018.

care for the body, mind, heart, soul, and support environment. The well-designed rehab plan includes actions which address each of these care needs in connection with the path to well-being.

In the previous essays, I have covered a range of topics: freezing motions, deep fatigue, mindfulness, terror management, lightness of being, and the importance of showing compassion and gratitude. The essays reflect my personal rehab plan, and they illustrate the diversity of domains that need to be addressed when taking the CHRONDI Creed into battle against a chronic disease. It is a tough battle! We need all the armor and weapons available.

It has taken me close to a decade to arrive at a rehab plan that works for my life with Parkinson's. There has been a lot of trial and error, many consults with professionals, and much research. The plan is not a static thing. It is always getting tweaked to keep ahead (or keep up!) with the changing demands of the chronic disease. The hardest thing for me has been to keep on the middle path, to not get too serious (intense, righteous) and yet not too flippant (not caring, lost in the clouds). The middle path is also about monitoring actions in all realms (body, mind, heart, soul, environment) to keep an even balance in thought and action. The middle way is about using just the proper amount of action applied to any situation and, as a result, getting back just the right consequences. The balance of the middle way can be built into the design of a rehab plan, and in doing so, aid the path toward well-being.

Every rehab plan is individually tailored, and the more closely it can match the needs of the individual, the more likely it is to be successful. But this can be a difficult goal to achieve. If you are a strong self-advocate, as I am, then there are many times of self-reflection and examination behind matching the rehab plan to personal needs.

If you are a caregiver, then the question that needs to be

continually revisited is, "How well do I know this person and his/her needs?" Truly walking in another's shoes, and having evidence that this has been accomplished, can reveal a person's true needs. There are varying degrees of empathy, and it takes skill to understand them and apply them. Empathy, and compassion, are the best tools to help arrive at the true needs of another. The mindset of the compassionate warrior is an important part of designing successful rehab plans.

It is hard work to design a detailed, individually tailored rehab plan. It is also challenging to put that plan into action, learn from it, tweak it repeatedly, and come up with an improved version. The opportunity for well-being to be present does not fall from a tree – we pick it when it is most ripe.

Others' Support within the Compassion Space

The O in the CHRONDI Creed stands for *Others* – the other people around us that support us, teach us, love us, pray for us, and provide care. Other people can also provide a mirror that helps us see how they perceive our actions. If we can objectively view this reflection, we can gain wisdom about the consequences of our actions, and then make informed choices that will affect how we interact with others. The relationships we have with other people provide a foundation of support seen clearly within the compassion space (see diagram below).

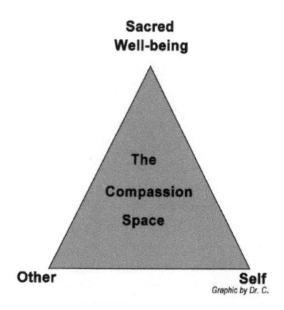

Sacred
Well-being

The

Compassion

Space

Other   Self

Graphic by Dr. C.

Columnist Sherri Woodbridge at *Parkinson's News Today* writes about relationships while dealing with PD,[36] saying that we need to consciously put the effort in to keeping that relationship magic alive and to seek help with relationship issues rather than trying to ignore them. It takes work to keep relationships healthy and growth-promoting. We never put our foot in the stream of life the same way twice – our lives constantly change, and our relationships need adjusting along with these changes.

Growth-promoting relationships with others happen within what I called the compassion space.[37] It is a shared space between self and the other and the possibility of well-being. There is also movement that takes place within this

---

[36] "Intimacy Can Be Challenging with Parkinson's Disease." by Sherri Woodbridge, "Journeying Through Parkinson's Disease," Published on Parkinson's News Today, February 6, 2019

[37] "Seeking the Soul of Life: A quest of compassion and finding our 'true self' in the midst of a hectic world," (Introduction) by Dr. C. at www.DrC.life

space. Reaching out to the other and then retreating to self (the "seek to get closer" and then later "push the person away") is one of the most common relationship dances. A similar dance happens when seeking to help someone toward well-being or to receive help from another with your own well-being. It is a dance of getting closer to well-being and then retreating from the experience. I have termed this compassion space resistance, and it is the main source of compassion fatigue.

Compassion fatigue does not arise from successful compassion.[38] Successful compassion leaves one with more energy than it takes, whereas compassion space resistance can be very draining and lead to caregiver burnout. When your life-long partner has a chronic illness, all you want to do is help move your partner towards a place with less suffering. But if the day has arguments about not following the rehab plan, or a lack of motivation to take personal responsibility for his/her half of the journey toward well-being, then the day is filled with resistance, and it can be exhausting.

Successful movement within the compassion space involves a shift toward well-being. When the self and the other are in the compassion space where this shift occurs, they experience a special type of growth-promoting relationship. It is called the "healing relationship." The healing relationship is often interpreted as sacred, as a gift, and something which is allowed, not demanded. Once the healing relationship is experienced, then the shift toward well-being becomes a stepping-stone both use in their own journeys toward maintaining a higher quality of life. The self then becomes a witness stepping-stone, saying things like, "Remember I was there with you." Then, as witness, asks the other person to

---

[38] Abendroth, Maryann and Flannery, Jeanne. "Predicting the Risk of Compassion Fatigue: A Study of Hospice Nurses." *Journal of Hospice and Palliative Nursing*, Vol. 8, No. 6, November/December 2006.

recall how much better she/he felt after the event. This witnessing happens within a different type of relationship, one called the "support relationship." The support relationship includes discussions on how the person can find his/her personal path to well-being.

Growth-promoting relationships involve entering the compassion space, in the roles of self and other. If we can understand the dance that takes place inside that space (the dance where the relationship changes from healing, to support, to resistance, and back again), then we can see our own path to well-being more clearly. Growth-promoting relationships are fundamental to success in the battle against a chronic disease. Healthy relationships depend upon the successful communication of our needs to each other. If you are waiting for the other person to read your mind and know what you need, then you are going to be disappointed. So much suffering in the world happens when people do not enter the compassion space, but instead throw words at each other from inside their personally constructed self-protection bubbles. We think we are safe inside our self-bubble. But the problem is that we can't really hear the needs of the other when inside that environment. If we can't hear the needs of the others in our lives, then it is difficult to have growth-promoting relationships.

Caregivers in our lives need our attention and compassion.[39] Others in our lives mirror ourselves and support our battle against a chronic illness. Use of the compassion space helps individual needs to be expressed and heard more accurately. It takes practice moving around in the compassion space with adept skill. The CHRONDI elements help with this practice.

---

[39] "Caregivers Need Attention, Too." Sherri Woodbridge, "Journeying Through Parkinson's Disease." Published on Parkinson's News Today, February 11, 2019.

Nature Walks and Gardening Improve Total Health

"Nature," the "N" of the CHRONDI Creed, has always been a part of my life. One doctor said to me, "Your strong history of exercise and nature has kept Parkinson's at bay." I was an avid hiker, cyclist, and rock collector. As I headed into my gray-hair years with PD, I moved from these activities to building and maintaining gardens around my home. I always felt healthier when gardening. In those early years of the disease, I did not know there is research[40] supporting that nature walks and gardening improve total health.

Human beings have been interacting with, and dependent on, nature as a means of survival for millennia. It has only been in the last several thousand years that we humans have migrated toward being city dwellers. Returning to our roots (pun intended) can have quite a few benefits. Living next to "green environments" has been shown to have both mental and physical health benefits.[41] Walks in parks, particularly when mindfulness is used, can have positive health benefits.[42] I can attest to the benefits of this practice, both personally and as a teacher of mindfulness. There are people who have trouble meditating while sitting. For many of them, a mindful walk in the woods can be helpful in quieting both mind and

---

[40] "Cultivate activity," Jeannine Stein. *Los Angeles Times*. January 5, 2009.

[41] Pearson, David G, and Tony Craig. "The great outdoors? Exploring the mental health benefits of natural environments." *Frontiers in psychology* vol. 5 1178. 21 Oct. 2014, doi:10.3389/fpsyg.2014.01178
See also "Massive Study Reveals Exposure to Nature Has Significant Health Benefits" by Joseph Mercola, MD., July 26, 2018. Organic Consumers Association.

[42] "Forest Bathing: A Retreat to Nature Can Boost Immunity and Mood," Allison Aubrey. *NPR Morning Edition*,
July 17, 2017.

body. Reconnecting to nature has total health benefits – and it doesn't have to take hours out of a busy life. Just minutes can make a difference,[43] particularly if done with mindfulness.

Humans have built sacred sites on, or near, places of great natural beauty. Experiencing the awe of natural beauty can leave a lasting effect, a change in body and mind. The wonder of nature is how our ancestors used the sacred sites to facilitate a doorway to the soul. Such doorways are nearly invisible when surrounded by hordes on the highways, multitudes straining the subway, and a spastic speed of technology stripping away our humanity. It is so easy to get lost in this modern culture, forgetting what was once intrinsically part of being human – the "nature" in human nature. Setting aside time each week to walk mindfully in a green environment is a first step to getting reconnected to our human nature.

Gardening takes more time than a stroll in the park, but there are additional physical benefits. Gardening is good exercise for people with PD, when adjusted for the severity of symptoms. I consider myself a "landscape painter" and gardening is my main form of exercise. Building garden beds and pathways is building a personal green space. I have a relationship with the plants in my garden. So much so, that I have moved plants, bulbs, and rootstock with me when changing homes. It could be construed as slightly crazy, but the plants were a physical reminder to me of times when I had more energy and fewer PD symptoms. Care for the garden and enjoying the beauty of blooms and foliage is a rich back-to-nature experience. For me, there is awe in the experience. Gardening has total health benefits that help me to manage the symptoms of a chronic disease.

---

[43] American Chemical Society. "In the green of health: Just 5 minutes of 'green exercise' optimal for good mental health." *ScienceDaily*, May 21, 2010.

The Death of Self – A Casualty of Chronic Disease

"Death" – the D in the CHRONDI Creed – refers more to the death of our self-identity than it does to physical death. As we battle through the long battle with a chronic disease, dealing with a gradual progression in symptoms, there is a loss of function. The stealing away of bits and pieces of both physical and mental function is touched upon in my essay about the "Disease Thief." The "Disease Thief" robs from us so many ways by which we know ourselves. It is a death of the self that is a casualty of chronic disease. It needs to be addressed with as much mindfulness as any other part of the creed for total health to be maintained at the highest level possible.

There is no manual for navigating through the death of self. I was educated in many ways to be prepared for it. Yet when it happened, I was shocked by the severity of its effects. PD gradually took from me those things which I identified as myself, those things I would proudly talk about when someone asked, "What do you do?" Below is the list of things stolen, roughly in chronological order:

- Field mineral specimen collecting since I was a teenager
- Professional field geologist
- Hiking and exploring rugged terrain
- Clinical counseling work
- Professor of counseling and geology

The time and money spent on four college degrees is behind all the years of experience expressed in the above list. Now all are casualties of a chronic disease. It is the death of self.

Looking in the mirror, past the gray hair and crevasses of age, deep into multicolored eyes, I find nothing that I remembered as me. The self I was knew was gone – dead! I was sitting in a void, a life without meaning, nothing of familiarity. From my clinical work, I knew that people get lost when this happens. It can be quite difficult to find the way back. I also knew something about this journey from mystical teachings,[44] but knowing and living through it personally are two different things. Somehow, I had to find my way out. I had to heal from the death of self.

The stages of grief can be applied to healing from the death of self. Work by Elisabeth Kubler-Ross[45] postulates that those experiencing grief go through a series of five emotions: denial, anger, bargaining, depression, and acceptance. I can clearly see that I touched upon each and every one. Denial and anger in the beginning – "I'm really OK" to "Why can't medical providers find the problem?" Bargaining to say if I only work harder physically, adjust my lifestyle, then maybe I can deal with all of this. I still have moments of depression. The losses seem to add up each year. As mentioned in the disease thief essay, terror management should be used as needed. It is important to have a support network through the process, including peers,[46] family,[47] and technology.[48]

Acceptance becomes more of a force these days. Both Mrs.

---

[44] Underhill, Evelyn. *The Cloud of Unknowing*. Edited from the British museum ms. Harl. 674, with an introduction by Evelyn Underhill. *A Book of Contemplation: Which Is Called The Cloud of Unknowing, in Which the Soul Is Oned with God.* London: J. M. Watkins, 1946.

[45] Kubler-Ross, Elisabeth and Kessler, David. *On Grief and Grieving: Finding the Meaning of Grief Through the Five Stages of Loss.* Scribner, 2014.

[46] Chronic Illness Alliance. "What is chronic illness peer support?" published on Chronicillness.org.au February 2019.

[47] AZoNetwork. "Family support critical for managing patients with chronic health problems." Published on www.news-medical.net, April 15, 2010.

[48] California Healthcare Foundation. "Using telephone support to manage chronic disease." June 2005.

Dr. C. and I work through that we must accept that schedules need to be adjusted, projects don't get the 110% attention we used to give, and family and friends may not understand what we face each day. There are still moments of regret and sadness. This is normal. The idea is to try to get to a level of understanding and accommodation for these restrictions. They are not failings – and that is an important thing to keep in mind. Through all the transitions, we are constantly redefining who we are – as individuals and in our relationships with each other and others. The next part of the CHRONDI Creed can be used to help with this acceptance and healing: the **I** (Identity) of the CHRONDI Creed.

A Healthy New Identity Helps when Battling a Chronic Disease

Identity – the "**I**" in the CHRONDI Creed – refers to the process of finding a health-fostering identity in the face of a chronic disease that has stolen things we loved to do and caused the death of self. When everything I loved to do and all forms of full-time employment were taken from me, all that was left was the time and energy I was putting into managing the disease. Dealing with a chronic disease consumes a huge amount of time. Conversations about me were now connected to the disease, including my own self-talk. Without even knowing how, and thinking I should know better, the disease had filled that void created by the death of self. The disease had become my identity and I hated it. I had to find a healthy new identity to help in my battle with chronic disease.

The search for identity, trying to "find yourself" is tied to some of those great philosophical questions: "What is the nature of human existence? Who am I?" I have been on this philosophical quest and I thought I had a handle on things, a strong identity of scientist, teacher, and healer. But when the models I used to play out these roles were stripped from me, I discovered that the intellectual writings provided a thin tether out of the dark void created by the death of self. The actions in my life, the conversations, did not match my identity roles of scientist, teacher, and healer. These well-known roles were close to the healthy identity I needed to succeed in my battle with a chronic disease. I need to bring these roles back into my life.

Aligning one's actions in life, the roles we take on, to match the true self is not an easy thing to do in the face of a chronic disease. It takes a commitment of personal resources, courage, and persistence to create new healthy roles to fill the void left after the death of self. It also helps to have support from peers, friends, and family. But most important – you need a fire in the belly, a passion, a purpose that brings meaning from these roles you will be creating. Then you need to do something every day that will move you one step closer to that purpose-driven life and a healthy identity matching the true self.

I started working on creating these new roles in 1999 when I left all that was my life, home, and career to pursue a Ph.D. – the second hardest challenge I have faced in my life. I also retrained myself to use the computer as a way of teaching, and for a tool in aiding scientific inquiry. In 2006, I applied those skills to a science research project which, after many years, has yielded new discoveries ready to share with the public. I taught myself to become a writer in the humanities by writing as often as time allowed. I also gained skills as a graphic artist, using the computer, and taught myself how to design a website. These skills – web design, writing, and graphic arts – helped me to reestablish the multimodal teacher role. In 2018, I became a column writer for BioNews Today, giving me the opportunity to put the multimodal teacher into action more frequently, hopefully as a role model. Recreating the roles of scientist and teacher, after the death of self, is ongoing for me. Every day, I make a commitment of time to these recreated healthy roles as part of building a new identity. It is hard work, but worth it.

The one part of my identity, which is still trapped in the void after the death of self, is my role of healer. It is a role that is closest to my true nature, my soul. I have testimonials from many people who state that their lives were changed through encounters with this healer role. I miss that contribution to the well-being of individuals and to the collective well-being of society. I don't know how to bring this role back into my life, but I am holding open the door to the possibility. Perhaps this book will serve to achieve that connection and offer my experiences to others as hope.

Finding the Courage to Face Life with a Chronic Disease using the CHRONDI Creed

The previous essays address the CHRONDI Creed, a plan anyone can put into place when seeking to live better with a chronic disease. The CHRONDI Creed is challenging to put in place as a way of life because it takes courage to face life honestly and to make the changes needed to move toward well-being. It takes courage to wake up every day with a chronic disease and to stand tall with the CHRONDI Creed as your action plan.

Life is about choices. Using the CHRONDI Creed is a choice. I could say to myself, "I am tired of having to do all this hard work." On bad days, that voice gets annoyingly loud. That voice was particularly loud while driving to my monthly doctor's visit for the other chronic disease I have – ocular histoplasmosis. It's an eye disease and I need chemical treatment injected in my eyes every month. This treatment is scary. Imagine watching a needle coming straight for your eyeball and then actually seeing the fluid being injected. Imagine the thoughts, the fears, and the discomfort doing this every month. I sign a waiver every time because of the risks involved with this treatment. Do I want to want to do this? Dumb question, right? But if I don't do it, then there is a chance that the disease will eventually take all my vision. It's a choice. I could choose not to do this treatment, but instead I choose to face this scary treatment every month. Courage is not the absence of fear but rather facing fear and doing what is health-promoting.

It takes courage to use the CHRONDI Creed as a way of living better with a chronic disease. CHRONDI stands for the following philosophy of chronic disease management:

C – Compassion: I will act compassionately toward others and find gentleness toward self.

H – Happiness: I will seek the inner bliss of happiness that is not material in nature.

R – Rehabilitation: I will apply courage and mindfulness to a total health rehabilitation plan.

O – Others: I will genuinely communicate to others my experiences and maintain an attitude of gratitude for their help.

N – Nature: I will take time to embrace nature and all its beauty, which may include gardening, walking, sitting in the quiet.

D – Death: I will find the courage to face the terror of the "death of self" (loss) and not let it control me.

I – Individuality: I will continue to express my individuality, and my purpose, beyond the disease.

The CHRONDI Creed is a series of self-affirming statements. I start each day with these statements and have been doing so for years. They have become my inner dialog – most of the time – to replace all the negative, sometimes nasty, inner noise. Keeping that negative noise down to a level of minimal impact is an especially important part of my personal plan for well-being.

Choosing to live by the CHRONDI Creed is not quite as daunting as having a needle stuck in your eye, but it is still something which takes a strong dose of courage. It takes courage to look honestly at your life and ask, "Am I living by this creed?" I have found that the CHRONDI Creed gives me more strength, helps me to have more courage, and adds to my quality of life while living with a chronic disease. I am always looking for ways to live the creed more completely.

My Partner has a Chronic Disease Also – The C.H.R.O.N.D.I. Creed Helps Us

The literature contains many articles that talk about caregivers supporting a person with a chronic illness, and that caregiver is usually the spouse or partner. But what is it like when both people in the relationship have a chronic disease? There is a lot less information out there about this predicament and what people can do under these circumstances to maintain a high quality of life. Mrs. Dr. C. and I have found that the CHRONDI creed helps us.

Seventy-five percent (75%) of marriages where one partner has a chronic illness end up in divorce. There is also a high degree of stress,[49] burnout,[50] and mental health issues.[51]

---

[49] "I have Parkinson's — and my wife is its invisible victim." Opinions. Don Riggenbach, *The Washington Post*, published March 4, 2016.

[50] "Caregiver Burnout: When Someone You Love Is Chronically Ill." Laura Reagan, LCSW-C, Posttraumatic Stress / Trauma Topic Expert Contributor, published on GoodTherapy.org, March 26, 2014.

[51] Savage, Sally and Bailey, Susan. 2004. "The impact of caring on caregivers' mental health: a review of the literature." *Australian Health Review*, Vol. 27, No. 1, pp. 103-109.

This has serious impacts on the health of the family.[52] Other writers have helpful suggestions on how to limit the negative relationship effects of a chronic disease, such as working through frustration,[53] and steps to use when there is irritability.[54] There are also good sources that provide a literature review of self-care,[55] a review of chronic illness as it overlaps with aging and elder issues,[56] and suggestions for information on caregiving. This information is useful, and it can be applied to the dueling chronic disease dilemma, but I have found that few articles accurately articulate the chaos that happens.

For us, Mrs. Dr. C. has had to take on much of the communication between us, providers, family, and friends. She is the only one able to drive, given my eye condition. She is a partner in many of our shared projects, contributing her insight and skills to helping create meaningful contributions in society. But due to her medical conditions, her physical resources have become more limited. She assures me that my recovery time from a three-hour drive is the same as hers. We

---

[52] Holmes, Ann M. and Partha, Deb. "The Effect of Chronic Illness on the Psychological Health of Family Members." *The Journal of Mental Health Policy and Economics* 6 (2003), 13-22.

[47] Caregiveraction.org. Caregiver Action Network is the nation's leading family caregiver organization working to improve the quality of life for the more than 90 million Americans who care for loved ones with chronic conditions, disabilities, disease, or the frailties of old age. CAN (the National Family Caregivers Association) is a non-profit organization providing education, peer support, and resources to family caregivers across the country free of charge.

[54] "The Grouch and T.O.O.T.S.: Dealing with Irritability." Dr. C. in Possibilities with Parkinson's, Parkinson's News Today, November 2, 2018.

[55] Ausili, Davide et. al. "A literature review on self-care of chronic illness: definition, assessment and related outcomes." *Professioni Infermieristiche*, Vol. 67, n.3, Luglio - Settembre pgs. 180-189.

[56] Rolland, John S., M.D. "Chronic Illness and the Life Cycle: A Conceptual Framework." *Family Process* 26:203-221, 1987.

both "crash" after long hours of driving, necessary to obtain medication or attend medical appointments or even to visit family. We schedule communal naps and let the errands or chores wait another day. Fortunately, we are both minimalists in our enjoyment of personal space. Clutter or disarray in our home diverts our attention. If I can help by taking out the garbage, I do it. If I can't manage to do a chore, then there are no repercussions from Mrs. Dr. C. It is a give and take – much of what needs to get done does get done. It just takes us both a bit longer.

If both people in the relationship must deal with their own chronic illness and then also be available and accessible to help their mate with their issues, chaos ensues. There is just no way around it – couples argue and fight. It's made worse when both have a chronic disease, with two people having illness issues and needs that must be met. It's a swirling storm that you either decide to travel through together, or you decide to each go your own separate ways. Mrs. Dr. C. and I have decided to make a commitment[57] to doing whatever needs to be done to make the journey easier and healthier for both. This is where the CHRONDI creed comes into play.

Compassion (C-CHRONDI) is the foundation for success, taking the time to hear each other's needs and respond with a gentle heart. Many of these needs fit into the care demands of disease management (R-CHRONDI), but relationship health must include more than the dueling illnesses. There needs to be times of shared happiness (H-CHRONDI), walks together embracing nature (N-CHRONDI), and supporting each other with the development of identities separate from the illness (I-CHRONDI). There is a positive side to both people having a chronic illness in that both are experiencing loss of function

[57] "My Spouse Has Parkinson's Disease, So I'm Going Out." Sherri Woodbridge in Journeying through Parkinson's Disease, Parkinson's News Today, February 19, 2018.

(D-CHRONDI) and both benefit from the support of others beyond the relationship (O-CHRONDI). We have agreed to put the CHRONDI creed in place as an umbrella to help weather the storms we encounter. It is a shared journey with each of us taking turns holding the umbrella against the fierce winds.

Our relationship has its rough times, fortunately not that often, but it also is a relationship filled with mutual interests, love, and a spiritual – soul – connection. We are first and foremost good friends. When the warranty on the body runs out and you can't get new parts anymore, it is these non-material qualities that bring strength to the relationship. We have always been each other's best friends, and even in the darkest of times, one of us shows up to hold the umbrella for the other one.

How Did Life Get So Busy? I Get So Overwhelmed!

I thought when I retired that I would have more time, not less. There just does not seem to be enough hours in the week to get done all the things I would like to do. If I push myself harder and longer, then I get fatigued and need more rest, which results in less time and defeats the purpose of pushing harder. I have a long list of things to do and I get overwhelmed looking at it, particularly when I am fatigued. This is a battle I have been having for the last five years, and there are a few things that make it a little easier for me.

To give you some idea of what my seven-day week used to look like, this was my "to do" list, with average hours I would spend on task:

Task	Hours
Writing	20
Geology project	10

House and garden/Exercise	20
Family time	10
Chronic disease maintenance	15
Chores, mealtimes	15
Play and relax time	20
Sleep	60
Total	170

A seven-day week has 168 available hours. I was already overbooked, and I haven't included several projects that are on my waiting to-do list. Last, but not least, are the requests for my professional services. This can take the form of a request for a paper or a presentation. When these requests come in, something on the above list had to change and I often got overwhelmed.

Being overwhelmed defeats the goal of finding more time to get things done because the emotional confusion puts a halt to effective project engagement. The way out of being so busy and feeling overwhelmed is to put into place some form of time management. The first thing is to realize how much time your chronic disease consumes each week. There are lots of ways this happens, and flexibility is crucial. The second thing is to block out the time that you need for those things that add to your well-being – like sleep, exercise, meals, and family. But, if you are like me with lots of irons in the fire, you may have a full list of things that require your time. So, it comes down to making choices, priorities, and sometimes I have to say "no" to people. Time is a resource that can be thought of like water in the well. You can only dip into the well a limited number of times before the well needs time to replenish. I also spend my time in concentrated blocks of three to four hours. This allows me to avoid distractions and to also reallocate those blocks when something unexpected comes up (and it always does!). I also have a partner who takes on much of the work that I can no longer physically do, which frees up time. Delegation, when you can, is a good time management strategy, along with simply asking someone for assistance, which can be difficult.

There are resources to help with time management skills and here are a few:

1) Time management skills book that looks at multiple life demands on our time.[58]
2) A thirty-minute audiobook talk with clear tips on time management.[59]
3) TED talk on time management.[60]
4) Columnists offer time management tips[61] and time management apps.[62]

Years after writing this piece, and progressing further with the disease, the time spent managing the illness has become a full-time job. I never know for sure when I'm going to have a bad day, so scheduling my time to meet with the outside world becomes quite difficult. In my own home, I can take breaks from my research and writing, and rest whenever needed. I look forward to good days and lucid moments when I can concentrate and communicate clearly. I don't force myself through the bad days like I used to. I just can't afford it anymore, but fortunately there still enough good days and lucid moments to continue writing.

---

[58] Davis, Russell. *Time Management: How to Achieve Work-Life Balance, Accomplish Goals, and Live a Happy Life.* Createspace Independent Publishing Platform, April 2017

[59] Greshes, Warren. *Time Management Skills that Work.* Audiobooks.com, December 2011.

[60] "How to gain control of your free time." Presented by Laura Vanderkam on Webcast, *TEDWomen 2016* | October 2016.

[61] "10 Tips for a 'Common Sense Approach' to Life with a Chronic Illness." Wendy Henderson in Social Clips, Parkinson's News Today, December 20, 2017.

[62] "6 of the Best Apps for Chronic Illness Management." Wendy Henderson in Social Clips, Parkinson's News Today, January 3, 2018.

Can You Hear Me Now?

Over the many years of living with a chronic illness, I have seen many health-care providers. Some were good and others, not so good. If I walked away from a meeting with a provider feeling like I wasn't heard and wanting to shout, "Can you hear me now?" then the provider wasn't a good match for me. Empathy (being heard by the provider) is deeply important to me and is a part of my quality health-care plan.

Over the past several decades, my research has focused on understanding the characteristics of a special relationship between patient and health-care provider that I call the healing relationship.[63] It is a therapeutic relationship which promotes patient well-being. Clinical empathy is a crucial part of this relationship. When the relationship functions well, the patient doesn't ask in desperation, "Can you hear me now?" The patient instead walks away from the relationship with a sense of being heard and understood. Along with that is a sense of trust in the provider and the treatment plan offered. This can then lead to a greater treatment compliance, a higher quality of health care, and better treatment outcomes.[64]

The healing relationship is not just something academic for me. It is something practiced. With retirement and the chronic illness, I had thought the skill had become too rusty to use, like an old pair of scissors left outdoors too long, and no longer retaining utility. But I had experiences in one week that surprised me with encounters where all three people asked for the healing relationship to happen. These three people had very traumatic events in their lives and all three needed solace.

---

[63] "Others Provide Support and a Mirror Within the 'Compassion Space.'" Dr. C. in Possibilities with Parkinson's, Parkinson's News Today, March 8, 2019.

[64] Halpern, Jodi. "What is clinical empathy?" *Journal of general internal medicine* vol. 18,8 (2003): 670-4. doi:10.1046/j.1525-1497.2003.21017.

Solace isn't handing them a chocolate chip cookie, saying, "I'm sorry you had to go through that. Here, take this. It will make you feel better." Solace happens through empathy, along with compassion, a type of *Tonglen* practice.[65] It is a sacred relationship in the sense that it is held with reverence and humility and never sought but always allowed. I thought I had lost this and am so incredibly grateful to be shown that I had not.

The health-care provider is there to meet the health-care needs of the patient. Those needs can only be accurately met when they are fully known. At times we, as patients, need to educate our providers.[66] There needs to be a shared dialog within the patient-provider relationship aimed at promoting well-being.[67] The characteristics of the healing relationship help the provider to acquire knowledge about the needs of the patient, while at the same time, developing a relationship of trust. When wisdom is added, compassion happens. Quality health care can occur. The healing relationship is not a new thing. Healers, doctors, nurses, and other health-care providers have been writing about it for the past few decades. They have been calling for a need to be filled within the practice of health care – to bring this art of healing back into health care. They may use the term "patient-centered care."

Medical care needs to be non-judgmental. The provider cannot provide quality care if he or she disparages the patient's evaluation of their disease. This is not to say the

---

[65] Chodron, Pema. *Good Medicine: How to Turn Pain into Compassion with Tonglen Meditation*. Audiobook. Sounds True, Incorporated, March 2001.

[66] "Educating the Educated About Parkinson's Disease." Sherri Woodbridge in Journeying through Parkinson's, Parkinson's News Today, February 27, 2019.

[67] Pieterse, AH, Stiggelbout, AM, Montori, VM. "Shared Decision Making and the Importance of Time." *JAMA*. 2019;322(1):25–26. doi:10.1001/jama.2019.3785

patient is always right. But the provider needs to be aware of the stress, frustration, and fear that the patient faces every day. These emotions will often cloud over a presentation. I've been known to present as a patient who "has it all under control." Clearly I don't. But the provider also needs to recognize that this is a form of self-identity. It's not a delusion. It's difficult to admit that the body and mind may be failing. Provider sensitivity to these emotions can help – lack of sensitivity can hinder.

Patients will want to scream, "Can you hear me now?" when the health-care provider seems not to be listening or seems to be absent of empathy. It is deeply frustrating not to be heard, because it leads to misunderstanding and health-care needs that are not met.[68] Fortunately, there are many health-care providers who do have empathy and compassion.[69] Finding those providers and incorporating them into your treatment team is a positive step toward personal well-being.

It's Not Just the Parkinson's Disease

In the essay on courage, I mentioned an eye disease that I have for which I receive monthly eye injections. Yes, you read that correctly. I get a needle in my eye. Actually, I get two needles, as one injection contains the additional anesthetic medicine after the topical application of numbing agent and the second injection contains the chemotherapy. The disease is unstable and progressive. Treatment is not the same thing as a cure. My providers do their best to keep things under

---

[68] Kong, Herbert Ho Ping and Posner, Michael. *The Art of Medicine: Healing and the Limits of Technology*. ECW Press, July 1, 2014.
[69] Lown, Bernard. *The Lost Art of Healing: Practicing Compassion in Medicine*. Ballantine Books; Reprint edition, February 2, 1999.

control. Unfortunately, I had a dramatic decompensation which has left me legally blind.

It's not the Parkinson's disease alone that makes life difficult, but rather all the other medical "stuff" that gets thrown on top of it. The loss of vision makes it much more difficult to do the quality columns I am so fond of writing for my readers. It's hard to adjust when such events hit unexpectedly and steal away another part of my self-identity.

Having been through other traumatic events in my life (and counseled others through traumatic injury), I know there is a process. There is a grieving process that Elizabeth Kubler-Ross describes.[70] There is also a recovery process. Often, not all is going to be as bad during the healing process as it initially appears. There is a flood of emotions which need to be taken in, understood, processed, and then let go so that the healing may continue. There is the time needed to make life adjustments to the effects of the physical trauma. All of this takes time, patience, and a gentleness with myself.

The first emotions I work through are anger: "*Why me? It's not fair!*" Then comes the self-pity: "*This is too hard. I just can't handle it. I wish someone would come and make it all better.*" Anger is a normal response. But anger and I just don't do well together. I can easily become the Grouch (see essay "The Grouch and T.O.O.T.S. – Dealing with Irritability").

I am an ugly Grouch, mostly because of what I call "spilling out behavior." It's been a bad day and the anger needs to go somewhere, so it spills out on those closest to me. Talk about not fair! I have way too many verbal skills to get into acrimonious word fights with those I care about. Self-pity also spills out on to all of those around me.

We may not realize it, but walking around with that dark cloud overhead casts a dark shadow on those closest to us.

---

[70] "The Five Stages of Grief: An Examination of the Kubler-Ross Model." Christina Gregory, Ph.D. on PsyCom.net, updated September 23, 2020.

Clinging to the hope that someone will save us from our own fate if we just whimper and whine loud enough does nothing but create more suffering. The choice then is to accept that something bad happened and that is just the way it is. Time to pull it together and attack the new challenges.

Don't get me wrong. I am not saying I feel all rosy and chipper about what has happened. I am upset, constantly reminded of the situation. Every time I open my eyes, I am forced to face head-on what has happened. If I let the emotions overwhelm me, I can't move forward. If I can't move forward, then my self-identity is headed for extinction. The choice is to accept the fact that something bad has happened and it is time to figure out how to deal with it.

Part of figuring out how to deal with a dramatic loss of vision (and its impact on my PD) will involve all those changes and adaptations to maintain a high quality of life. This new journey has just begun. At this point, I needed to take a short break while I completed the medical procedures to stave off further vision loss. Then I had to put into place any adaptations necessary to learn new techniques for using the computer screen, using pen and paper, and exploring other adaptive equipment. PD had to take a back seat to all of this.

To their credit, the Veterans Administration Low Vision Clinic staff rose to the challenge. I cannot express my gratitude in their efforts to find accommodations. I have specially lined paper to direct my scrawling handwriting. They found a hand-held magnifying glass that lets me read most of the fine print on labels or on the computer. Above all, they were caring and compassionate to me, understanding not only the challenges of loss of vision, but what it means in terms of that impact on Parkinson's. They understand when I report breaking sunglasses because I dropped them while trying to hold on to pieces of paper and just couldn't coordinate the whole thing with fluid motions. No chastisement for my lack of manual incoordination. Now, if we could figure out a better way for me to use those infernal cash card machines at the grocery store!

Additionally, I want to acknowledge that during that time, I had support from all my readers, editors, writers, and staff at BioNews Services for their kind words of support and encouragement. I reminded them that even in the face of adversity, in the esteemed words of the former governor of California, "I'll be back!"

Compassionate Support and Wellness

It was rough going with acquiring the "legally blind" diagnosis on top of Parkinson's. Part of the reason I was able to return to column writing so soon was because of the compassionate support I received that was freely given.[71] It made a big difference in my life. The compassionate support bolstered my wellness program and gave me the added strength I needed to move forward.

People speak of wellness as some sort of bonus from doing something because it's "good for you." Eat vegetables or walk 10,000 steps a day because they are "good for you." But doing suggested beneficial acts is not the only factor in the wellness process. The wellness that comes from compassionate support is more than that. When support is given in a truly compassionate way, it reflects not only on the act of support, but on the possibility that we can be a "better self." It doesn't matter how bad things appear, because compassionate

[71] Ghorbani Saeedian R, Nagyova I, Krokavcova M, Skorvanek M, Rosenberger J, Gdovinova Z, Groothoff JW, van Dijk JP. "The role of social support in anxiety and depression among Parkinson's disease patients."
Disability Rehabilitation. 2014;36(24): 2044-9. doi: 10.3109/09638288.2014.886727.
Epub Feb 18, 2014.

support can make things better. It works.

There are lots of ways to block off connecting to the compassion others offer. Sometimes it seems easier to give than to receive. While I was grappling with the vision loss that month, I didn't want to go to the local PD support group. I felt like a failure, to everyone and to myself. The pain and suffering I was going through created a wall between me and the rest of the world.[72] My partner of almost 50 years, Mrs. Dr. C., convinced me to go. Allowing myself to be vulnerable, to let down those walls and enjoy the support group, also allowed me to feel this potential for the betterment of mankind. I connected to that for my personal well-being.[73] Moaning about how terrible I feel doesn't get me anywhere. I am trying to focus on the here and now, to keep a positive attitude about tomorrow.

Several years ago, Mrs. Dr. C. and I moved to a new house that was more ADA accessible, changed career focus, re-built our caregiver/social network, and dealt with each untoward event that has popped up along the way. Mrs. Dr. C. walked with me through all of this while having her own medical issues.[74] Often fatigued from a particularly insidious infection of Lyme disease and occasionally overwhelmed by the demands of side effects both of treatment and disease, she fought hard to improve our quality of life. She made sure I

[72] Jane Simpson, Katrina Haines, Godwin Lekwuwa, John Wardle, and Trevor Crawford. "Social support and psychological outcome in people with Parkinson's disease: Evidence for a specific pattern of associations." *British Journal of Clinical Psychology* (2006), 45, 585–590 q 2006, The British Psychological Society.

[73] "Better Social Support Linked to More Positive Living Experience, Study Shows." Marisa Wexler, published on Parkinson's News Today, April 11, 2019.

[74] Lindsay H. Ryan, Wylie H. Wan, and Jacqui Smith. "Spousal social support and strain: impacts on health in older couples." *J Behav Med.* 2014 Dec; 37(6): 1108–1117. Published online 2014 Mar 13. doi: 10.1007/s10865-014-9561-x

didn't stray too far from our commitment to each other and to rehabilitation. She advocated a strong "no-nonsense" encouragement and was firm about the importance of continuing to engage in life. She is also probably the only person in my life who can interpret my email typographic errors and the scrawling handwritten notes. But as she says, "I read doctors' handwriting for years... this isn't much different!"

There is much research that lends credence to this idea that humans helping one another, sharing in the process of compassionate support, can make a difference in wellness. A recent study showed a stronger purpose in life was associated with lower all-cause mortality. Several interventions have been clinically reviewed including well-being therapy, demonstrating improvements in purpose in life, quality of life, and various health outcomes.[75]

The O in CHRONDI is for Others. It speaks to the interconnectedness we have with each other, connections that can help with our wellness. This is not about some supernatural phenomena or "butterfly effect." Rather, it is about a human relationship phenomenon that exists to share a flow moment in time. It is the experience of gratification after allowing ourselves to embrace the compassion being given. The compassion given and received is a fundamental part of the relationship I call the healing relationship, which is available on the Dr C website.[76]

There can be resistance to the healing relationship that is connected to compassionate support. Connectedness doesn't usurp identity. I sit on the island of individuality often. The

---

[75] Aliya Alimujiang, MPH, Ashley Wiensch, MPH ; Jonathan Boss, MS, et al. "Association Between Life Purpose and Mortality Among US Adults Older Than 50 Years." *JAMA Network Open.* 2019;2(5):e194270. doi:10.1001/jamanetworkopen.2019.4270
[76] www.DrC.life

idea of self has special meaning for me: the "I" in CHRONDI. When it comes to wellness, that island is the last place I want to be.

Are We There Yet?

How do I know when I'm getting well? There's that child's voice yelling from the back seat of the car reminding me that time waits for no man. I would like to say, "Hey, we are almost there?" but I am not sure what "there" looks like. Perhaps getting well is just "feeling like your old self again." Saying that as a way of describing a wellness process doesn't clearly describe the phenomena occurring during the process of getting well. What it does communicate is the idea that getting well is something people want to experience. People do hope to return to an experience of their "old self" again. The recent medical issue with my eyes, along with PD, has forced me into a different perspective. While I can't give the answer I'd like to the child's demand, "Are we there yet?" I can answer, "The GPS has us right on track."

We each have our own definition of wellness. We know that sense of feeling "like my old self." It's a map showing us a way from our current state to one where we feel better. There are signposts on the map that point us toward wellness. How we have come to understand these signs is likely to be as varied as PD. It is easy at any point in life to become so overwhelmed that it seems as if there are no signposts. And sometimes, no map. I flail about for a while, get all emotional. With the help from family and friends, I return to my old self, a shift toward wellness. I constantly remind myself that there is an atlas. To believe anything else means to disbelieve in the holistic scientific philosophy that is the foundation of "Dr. C." It's a fight to push rational thoughts over emotion to regulate the emotional effects following an injury. It is hard to do, but the wellness map is worth the effort. Regulation of emotion is part of my wellness map.

I have heard, "If you have met a person with PD, then you have met one person with PD." PD expresses itself uniquely in each of our lives. In the same way, our map of wellness – or way of living well with PD – is specific to our own way of experiencing the world. Even though PD is slightly different for everyone, there are some shared phenomena. For example: motor control problems, change in cognitive performance, and experiencing "off and on" periods are just a few commonalities. It's the shared phenomena that helps to provide a shared language for communication about not only PD, but also about our journey using the map of wellness.

One of the first things I do when serious injury happens to me (and I feel upset and/or confused) is to simplify live. I need time to heal. I need to make time in life to simplify the demands on my time to free up my schedule for wellness. It must be a conscious decision to put more time into wellness and to do so with a committed resilience and a sacred intent. I agree to do what I know I need to do for myself to heal. I am not talking about some selfish dive into a pint of Ben and Jerry's ice cream without offering to buy a pint for your partner. Healing while taking care of others is not only possible, but also compatible. The sense of personal sacred healing space is a space without distraction. It is focused on a state of being which best supports the healing needs at that interconnected moment. Getting back to that space is my current journey. This is where I think practice has helped and this is part of my wellness map.

I have written about the CHRONDI Creed and the compassionate warrior's mental frame. My map includes such a mental frame. Ideally, it is not angry. Rather, it is filled with energy that can be directed as needed by a wellness warrior in terms of preparations, resilience, and a sacred intent. The idea that sacred intent is connected to our personal wellness journey is not as strange as it might seem. For millennia, we humans have held a great reverence for those who could facilitate the well-being of the tribe members.[77] Sacred is not the same as religious. It is more about a reverence for the process surrounding the attainment of well-being. I have reverence for the beauty of science and for the spiritual aspects of who we are as humans. For me, there is so much intertwining to find a peaceful coexistence between the mystic side and the scientific side. In writing about wellness, I can't let go of one side in favor of the other. It is going to be a challenge to blend the two into a new view.

Wellness: Finding the Way to Well-being

Wellness is the map of actions and thoughts we use to guide us toward a higher quality of life, a life with more moments experiencing well-being. Our wellness map is tailored to meet our individual needs and must be flexible and adaptable. Life is always throwing out curve balls. Human resilience[78] is connected to how well we can adapt our wellness map. I have Parkinson's, and I continually tweak the wellness map to the changing conditions of this progressive disease. The new onset of vision loss required more than tweaks. It required some major changes to the wellness map. Understanding the basic structure of a wellness map is helping me find my way to more moments of well-being.

---

[77] "An initial investigation into the possibility of advanced empathy – a description of the healing relationship," Ph.D. Thesis, W. David Hoisington, Syracuse University, 2003.

[78] Bonanno G.A. "Loss, trauma, and human resilience: have we underestimated the human capacity to thrive after extremely aversive events?." *American Psychol.* 2004 Jan; 59(1):20-8.

When making a wellness map, the process involves: 1) a design that meets individual needs; 2) accessing available resources; 3) implementation; and 4) follow up. A successful wellness map will utilize the resources available to the individual including support from other persons, personal strengths, and the person's history of well-being experiences. The wellness map will also need to be consciously implemented with compassion and sacred intent. Finally, there needs to be follow up where the success of the map is evaluated. These processes are all intertwined into a holistic view of wellness.

Few of us are professionally trained in all the complexities of human wellness. We need not only the knowledge of illnesses and available treatments, but also the wisdom about the efficacy of wellness possibilities. This means we require wellness mapmaking wisdom from the experts to keep our wellness map functioning to the highest degree possible. The process of choosing which experts to listen to, and then how to wisely incorporate their wisdom into our personal wellness plan, is tied into the science of human decision-making.

Each of us has individual wellness needs and our own decision-making processes used to design and implement our wellness map. The CHRONDI Creed contains the fundamental elements for building a PD wellness map. It doesn't address the process of upgrading one's personal map in the face of new trauma.

Vision loss affects PD in ways I am still understanding. Vision has been a big part of how I enjoyed the beauty and science of the world. Writing, science research, photography, artwork, flower gardens, and viewing the world with its multitude of colors and shapes provided me with hours of enjoyment. Loss of vision left me feeling disconnected from life. Things don't appear clear, as bright and beautiful as before. The pleasure once received from visual stimuli was not the same. I have a deeper understanding of how important "pleasure chemistry" and happiness are to the treatment of PD and the risks of either losing that or trying to artificially replace it. My new wellness map will take all of this into consideration.

There are days when there is no clear vision of what needs to be done (no pun intended). Shifting to the basics helps – exercise, eating well, quiet mind, and gratitude. It's a focus on healing, with reducing internal and external language about feeling sick. This doesn't mean I ignore the physical ailments and the treatments. It means that my disease treatments are wrapped up in a comforting blanket of wellness. Sometimes, fatigue hits hard and there isn't the energy to pursue wellness map making. Back to basics – rest, meditate, and let it go. There will be tomorrow. Build patience and compassion into the wellness map.

Redesigning a wellness map is about choosing wisely how to use time. Staying out of toxic thinking/acting and toxic environments. Spending more time engaged in wellness-related thoughts and actions, those having the greatest potential for leading to moments of well-being. It is a life focus on being well, not on complaining about suffering. One carves out a little piece of time from the large amount dedicated to thinking/acting in response to sickness, and then allocates that little block of time to wellness. The wellness map is built with a practice of thought and action that bolsters the healing process and helps hold open the door to more moments of well-being. It takes resilience, patience, and hard work to forge an improved wellness map, and it is never too late to start working on it.

Moments of Well-being and a Healing Perspective when Using the Wellness Map

A man walks into a store and asks for a map. The

storekeeper responds, *"We have lots of maps. Where are you going?"* The man snaps, *"Anywhere but here."* The shopkeeper says, *"Sorry. We don't have a map to 'Anywhere but Here.'"*

When first hit with the sudden loss of vision, I just wanted to escape. Anywhere was better than here. I thought I had lost my way to well-being because all I saw was a distorted view of life when viewed through my obscured vision. It seemed as if I had no wellness map. It took me a while to realize that there is no wellness map to "anywhere but here." A wellness map is used to help us move toward increased probability for well-being moments. The first step in that direction is to have a perspective which promotes healing. A well-being moment can be described as bliss,[79] flow,[80] mystical,[81] and healing.[82] A well-being moment is characterized by clear euphoria, awe, sense of time loss, a shift in perception, and wisdom. Well-being moments are holistic, touching mind, body, emotions, and soul. It is these characteristics which distinguishes them from artificial "feel good" moments. I define these "feel good" moments as fleeting, non-sustainable, and leaving behind the desire for more intense stimulation that has to be forced into existence. Well-being moments can permeate an individual's entire being. "Feel good," once past, leaves a feeling of emptiness. Think of the difference as experiencing sunshine warming you to the core (well-being) and the surge that you feel eating ice cream. The ice cream craving might return as quickly as it came. It will leave with only the thoughts of

---

[79] Campbell, Joseph. *The Power of Myth*. Anchor Books, Knopf Doubleday Publishing Group, 1991.

[80] Csikszentmihalyi, Mihaly. *Flow: The Psychology of Optimal Experience*. Harper Perennial Modern Classics, 2008.

[81] Eliade, Mircea. *Shamanism: Archaic techniques of ecstasy*. Princeton, NJ: Princeton University Press. 1974.

See also Underhill, Evelyn. *Mysticism: The nature and development of spiritual consciousness*. Reprint 1999, Boston: One World Publications.

[82] www.DrC.life

seeking more ice cream. Well-being will continue for a long time and can give rise to introspection and healing.

PD is a long, gradual, progressive disease. There are changes and losses. The CHRONDI Creed illustrates some of the changes I have made along the way to my wellness map. There were moments of the realization of loss – loss in my physical stamina, loss of my ability to work, loss of my coordination, and the loss of my ability to do things easily that I had enjoyed for many years. Many of the changes incorporated a shift in perspective.

Following the vision loss in combination with my PD, the very first tweak I made to my wellness map was to stop perseverating on the loss and shift to seeking wisdom. It is more than going past grief and accepting the loss. It is a shift of focus away from loss, disease, and suffering and on to what was gained in this new PD reality. The first tweak to the wellness map is shifting the perspective about the trauma. This is done to allow for more moments of well-being.

To some people, there is confusion about well-being. So much suffering is linked to chasing after the feel-good aspect of well-being. Some think that the fleeting moment of feeling good is all there is. They push to reach out and grasp (or purposefully try to create) that moment of rapture. Grasping the butterfly only destroys its wings. Not grasping helps allow wellness to unfold. Tweaks to a wellness map are aimed at opening the possibility for well-being moments to occur and hold open that possibility with compassion, lightness, and patience. There have been times when I lost a sense of well-being, or had trouble using my map, but shifting to a healing perspective helped me find my way back.

Do I have moments when the PD wears me down or makes me frustrated? Of course. Do I have moments when the vision loss feels like "just one more thing" to lose in my life? Absolutely. But each day is spent with the intent that I can continue to create my wellness map and walk towards a sense of well-being despite these challenges. Having PD and the vision loss does not make me less of a person – to myself, my family, my friends, or my contributions to the world at large. It's just a new way of seeing and interacting with the world to which I can adjust. I believe events are intertwined across time and space. This vision loss was connected to more of my life, including how I experienced PD, than I was willing (or perhaps able) to understand at the time. The shift in perspective helped me to understand the meaning of my experiences, decrease the angst, and increase the frequency of well-being moments.

Well-being moments cannot be forced to happen. Alternatively, we create a life, an inner relational space, which is more conducive to the occurrence of well-being moments. Learning how to wisely access a shift in perspective is an important part of living within that sacred relational space. Well-being moments are characteristically difficult to describe. Perhaps we can come together and share our experiences of these well-being moments in the face of PD, and in doing so, expand our collective understanding.

Shifting Perspective – Shifting Possibility

I hate exercise! Both pain and fatigue increase for me when I exercise. Pain and fatigue are disabling PD symptoms, and both trigger the fight-or-flight response that often manifests as the "Grouch." I have by no means come to a satisfying solution on exercising with PD pain and fatigue in a way that is easy, but I have found ways to shift my perspective. Shifting perspective opens the possibility of experiencing enjoyment from exercise.

One of the most important parts of a PD wellness map is exercise. But here's the catch – it's difficult to do with regularity[83] and at an intensity that will make a difference.[84] We know it works! Yet knowing what is good for wellness is not the same as doing it. Doing exercise, showing up three to four times a week, is difficult with all the chronic disease barriers. It's easy to feel defeated before even starting.

The way around this apparent Catch-22 is to shift one's perspective on exercise. The idea of shifting perspective in connection to wellness is about well-being moments. The shifted perspective needed with exercise is one that will get me off the sofa and into exercising. I am not getting off the sofa to do something I hate, but rather to do an enjoyable creative project which involves exercise – landscaping to produce gardens. It's a good exercise to keep the core strong and protect against falls.[85]

It takes a bit of perseverance to get into my work clothes, strap on the heavy work boots, find the hat, sunglasses, and then head out the door. Surveying the work ahead – sometimes a bit daunting – I start with light work to warm up. Walk, then shovel, maybe raking, before getting behind the wheelbarrow to move gravel or dirt from one location to another. Pause to hear the birds sing, marvel at the variety of flower blooms and fragrances. Pretty quickly, the world slips away, replaced by the Zen of gardening. My Fitbit reminds me if a medication time is coming up and keeps track of my heart rate. Lots of water breaks needed! Mrs. Dr. C. is checking on me. By the time two hours has passed, my work shirt is

---

[83] Oliveira de Carvalho, Alessandro, et al. "Physical Exercise For Parkinson's Disease: Clinical And Experimental Evidence." *Clinical practice and epidemiology in mental health: CP & EMH* vol. 14 89-98. 30 Mar. 2018, doi:10.2174/1745017901814010089

[84] Rosenthal, Liana S, and E Ray Dorsey. "The benefits of exercise in Parkinson disease." *JAMA neurology* vol. 70,2 (2013): 156-7. doi:10.1001/jamaneurol.2013.772

[85] "Trunk Exercises May Improve Balance in Parkinson's Disease, Study Finds." Catarina Silva, MSC, on Parkinson's News Today, March 20, 2019.

drenched with as much, if not more, sweat[86] than water I've consumed. In the Zen garden moments, the mind is free of the worries of PD and vision problems. That feeling remains with me, not as a false euphoria, but a deep-rooted sense of well-being.

There are many ways that shifting perspective can open wellness possibilities. A nurse shared a wonderful example. She was a smoker from her early teen years, and in her thirties, she decided to quit. Six months without a smoke and she said, "I had this memory of how much I enjoyed smoking." So, she bummed a cigarette and immediately got sick from her brief return to smoking. Recounting the event, she said, "I can remember the horrid feeling as clear today as if it just happened. I never had the urge to smoke again after that." She shifted her perspective from enjoying smoking to thinking of it as a horrid sickening experience. Shifting perspective opened the possibility of wellness.

There is research supporting the practice of shifting perspective in a way that promotes well-being. The placebo effect is believed to use a shift in perspective that results in an improvement in well-being.[87] Also, in many cases of "miracle" disease remission, a common theme is the patient's ability to shift perspective.[88] Reframing a problem can provide a new

---

[86] Swinn L., Schrag A., Viswanathan R., Bloem B.R., Lees A., Quinn N. "Sweating dysfunction in Parkinson's disease." *Movement Disorders.* 2003 Dec;18(12):1459-63. doi: 10.1002/mds.10586. PMID: 14673882.

[87] Linde, Klaus et al. "Placebo interventions, placebo effects and clinical practice." *Philosophical transactions of the Royal Society of London. Series B, Biological sciences* vol. 366,1572 (2011): 1905-12. doi:10.1098/rstb.2010.0383

See Also

Kaptchuk, Ted J. and Miller, Franklin G., Ph.D. "Placebo Effects in Medicine." *N Engl J Med* 2015; 373:8-9 DOI: 10.1056/NEJMp1504023

[88] Turner, Kelly A. *Radical Remission: Surviving Cancer Against All Odds.* Harper One; 1st edition (September 1, 2015).

perspective and lead to new solutions.[89] The ability to shift perspective may also improve our ability to adapt to stressful times and to become more resilient, and thus more open to new possibilities. The shifting of perception causes us to shift our focus to a new intention, a new possibility. I feared exercise because of the pain it would cause, and my intention was to avoid it. The shift in perception offered the new intention of enjoyment and the possibility of a beautiful garden along with a healthier body, despite the chronic disease limitations.

As the disease progresses, I find that the practice of shifting perspective is crucial to me living well with a failing body. I can't always get out to my garden. I can't always find the energy to do as much as I would like to do. My shift in perspective has to be, "It's OK to do what I can."

Managing Chronic Pain – Understanding a Shift in Perspective

Pain and suffering are not the same. An online search of "difference between pain and suffering" yields dozens of writers and practitioners extolling the benefits from this conceptualization. The repeated message is that pain is the physical experience connected to insult and injury, while suffering is the "story" we tell ourselves about the pain experience. Our total pain experience is the sum of physical pain and suffering, with each affecting each other. Shifting the perspective on chronic pain to one which understands the role of suffering in the total pain experience has helped to better

---

[89] "Reframing your thinking." Student Life and Learning Ground Floor, Building J, University of the Sunshine Coast, Maroochydore DC QLD 4558, Australia. https://www.usc.edu.au/media/3850/Reframing yourthinking.pdf

manage my chronic pain, a decrease in the occurrence of dysregulated emotions, and an overall improvement in well-being.

The difference between pain and suffering is an encyclopedic topic, having been the focus of writings since at least the time of the Buddha.[90] The focus here is on the mind/body link and how we can use that information to better manage chronic pain. The mind/body link as an attention-to-stimulus process was partially described in the essay on irritability. It's the process of pain stimulus (attention to the stimulus/feelings/thoughts), then recognizing body pain, addressing the pain in a therapeutic way, and back to start the process all over. It is a feedback loop that helps us in the face of danger. But as the feedback cycles out of control, then emotions often become unregulated and out of control. The spiraling loop can become a barrier to well-being. The experience of emotion dysregulation (see figure page 93) can disrupt and increase the pain, delay or inhibit feedback, demand the redirection of attention processes, and increase suffering.

The figure illustrates emotion dysregulation as an experience connected to exceeding one's emotion dysregulation threshold (EDT) due to increasing emotional intensity over time (dysregulation delay – DD). Once the threshold is crossed, there we experience emotional dysregulation (EDE). This is followed by a cooling of the emotion intensity (CD). In a sense, it is the process of "letting off steam" – but one that isn't always the best or effective way. Breaking through the threshold can ultimately result in destructive actions – to self or others.

---

[90] *Basics of Buddhism.*
https://www.pbs.org/edens/thailand/buddhism.htm

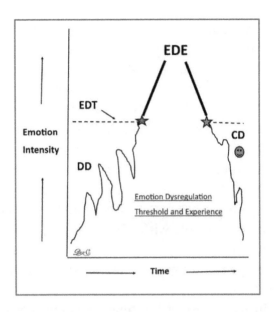

The goal is to reduce the intensity and duration of the EDE. This is where the shift in perception is applied. It is a shift from emotions getting out of control and feeling like we can't do anything about them to understanding that we can change the escalation. We can adopt the perception that we have some control over this dysregulation and that, given the nature of neural plasticity (if we exercise our conscious control over the processes behind emotion dysregulation), then there is the possibility of less intense dysregulation experiences and longer dysregulation delay times. This success can lead to less suffering and make it easier to manage chronic pain.

Pain is reported by many PD patients. "Among the different forms of PD-related pain, musculoskeletal pain is the most common form, accounting for 40%–90% of reported pain in PD patients. Individuals with Parkinson's disease frequently suffer from pain that interferes with their quality of life but may remain under-recognized and inadequately treated," according to a study published online in the *Journal of Neurology.*[91] I am one of them. I have good days and then there are those unbelievably bad days – the ugly days.

"We found pain to be highly frequent, quality of life-impairing but insufficiently and unsystematically treated," wrote first author Carsten Buhmann, M.D., of the University Medical Center, Hamburg-Eppendorf (Hamburg, Germany) and colleagues.[92] I have actually had providers tell me that Parkinson's patients do not experience pain from the disease.

When we live with Parkinson's disease (PD) and experience pain, we are not alone. **Chronic pain is twice as common among people with PD as it is in people without it.** In fact, more than **80%** of people with PD report experiencing pain and say it's their most troubling non-motor symptom.[93]

I am in pain most of the time. Crossing that threshold happens when I am having difficulty managing the pain and the connected feedback loop. If I add some additional stressor – emotional, physical, situational – then that feeds the emotional turmoil, and the threshold is crossed sooner. Accepting that I can do something about it and have the skills is the shift in perspective. It is a shift from being a servant to the whims of my emotions and their consequences to a presenting as a calm, centered being who seeks continued progress on his wellness map.

I am still learning and practicing techniques to help me

---

[91] Skogar, Orjan, and Johan Lokk. "Pain management in patients with Parkinson's disease: challenges and solutions." *Journal of multidisciplinary healthcare* vol. 9 469-479. 30 Sep. 2016, doi:10.2147/JMDH.S105857

[92] "Parkinson Disease: Pain Treatment" by Veronica Hackethal, MD, published on NeurologyLive.com, April 6, 2017.
See also: Buhmann C, et al. "Pain in Parkinson disease: a cross-sectional survey of its prevalence, specifics, and therapy." *J Neurol.* 2017 Feb 27.

[93] "Pain in Parkinson's Disease." Parkinson's Foundation. Parkinsons.org, 2018.

shift my perspective so that I can manage my chronic pain more successfully. Changing human practices are only as effective as the intent behind them. The shift in perspective allows us to firmly establish this proper intent.

Managing Chronic Pain: Applying a Shift in Perspective with The Pause Between

Pain attacks me every day and much of my time each day is set aside to manage it. Chronic pain management is now a significant part of my wellness map. The techniques used for pain management are rooted in 1) the conceptualization of total pain as suffering plus pain; 2) that a portion of that suffering is connected to dysregulated emotions; and 3) I know that it is possible for me to make positive changes that will reduce the amount of pain that I experience each day.

It is only recently that pain has become a daily experience, thus becoming the focus of my wellness map tweaking. The tweaking is a more focused attention on the **"pause between."** It is a mental, and often physical, pause before continuing to think or act to decrease the occurrence of dysregulated emotions and their consequences. Putting this in practice decreases suffering, reduces the frustrations I feel, and thus decreases my perception of pain.

Pain often triggers the fight/flight response which then triggers emotion. Emotions triggered by pain are followed by thought and often action. It is a feedback loop designed to keep us safe from danger. But the loop can spin almost out of control. To keep it from escalating, it is possible to insert a pause in the loop. This is a pause between pain and emotion, between emotion and thought, and/or between thought and action.

The pause between is first brought into focus through

knowing its possibility and directing attention to that possibility. This is a shift in perspective which says, "I can practice the pause between, and it will lower my pain." It is a shift in how the mind is used during the day. Wherever I decide to take my mind each day creates a path that is easier to take the next day. The brain likes familiar roads.

Sitting with the pause between takes daily practice. Maybe I should be grateful for the PD chronic pain reminding me of the importance of such practice. There are days when the PD chronic pain is draining – on all levels. There are times when no matter what I do, I can't sit in the pause between, but I believe in neural plasticity.[94] If I keep my brain practicing pain management, then it will become easier.

The success of this practicing is enhanced by the construction of a wellness map. The CHRONDI elements can serve this function. Techniques that help to quiet the mind, slow it down, are helpful in allowing more opportunities to sit in the pause between.

A mentor, something I have been for many students, can also help another to experience the pause between and arrive at a better understanding of the individual's resistance to sitting there. The pause is a suspended moment that is not filled with normal emotion, thought, or action. Judgement is suspended and focus is aimed at sitting in the pause between. It is very brief at first, but with practice, the pause between can become longer in duration and more easily accessible. The pause between is like a fork in the road. Choose which fork to take, with thought and action, and eventually with emotion. The pause between changes patterns of thought and action, decreasing the frequency of those contributing to suffering by choosing a different side of that fork in the road. The pause

[94] Sharma, Nikhil, et al. "Neural plasticity and its contribution to functional recovery." *Handbook of clinical neurology* vol. 110 (2013): 3-12. doi:10.1016/B978-0-444-52901-5.00001-0

gives us the time to walk down that new path beyond the fork, putting new patterns of thought and action in place. This helps to reduce suffering, and thus reduce pain.

There is a wide diversity of techniques one can apply to practice sitting in the pause between. Here are but a few:

- Divert your attention to other tasks, for example, reading book or playing a video game.
- Engage in physical exercise, a walk, or a bicycle ride.
- Get involved in a positive activity that brings with it meaning and purpose.
- Meditate.
- Talk to someone who can help.
- Use T.O.O.T.S. ("Time Out on The Spot"[95])
- Calmly, rationally, evaluate your choice of thoughts, and/or actions, and choose wisely.

I have used all of these, and still do. These techniques work better when I recognize and start first with the pause between with the goal of reducing personal suffering.

About Pain: Conversation with Neo

Bad pain day. Trying to keep my mind distracted. Perhaps a good show is on the television. Or maybe a movie. In a few hours, "off" cycle will kick in. Pain gets worse. Last medication before bed. Time to be quiet and contemplative, but this is squelched by the pain. Always murmuring, sometimes shouting, and always present. Finding sleep means I need to sit in the "pause between." I speak this mantra to myself:

You can do this - breathe in 1, 2. Breathe out 1, 2.
Let go and allow.

---

[95] "Psychology Tools: How to Take a 'Time Out'" by Kim Pratt, LCSW, published on HealthyPsych.com, January 11, 2014.

My mind will have nothing to do with this "pause between" nonsense.

Waving the imagined finger, my brain's neocortex, "Neo," interrupts and in rapid fashion says, "How's that to-do list coming? You're feeling like you didn't get much done today. Trying to make up for that by working on a new to-do list but having trouble focusing. This pain sure is annoying."

Neo is always intruding on my search for the pause between. He can be more annoying than the pain. I respond flatly, "Yeah, nothing new." I shift in bed to try to be more relaxed during my search for the pause between.

You can do this – breathe in 1, 2,3. Breathe out 1, 2,3.
Let go and allow.

Neo pokes a nerve cell. "Remember what the pain was like the other night? Whoo-ee, you were tossing and turning, and I felt like we were on a roller coaster!"

Night often starts with thrashing in bed. While I constantly switch positions to find comfort, the covers take on a life of their own, and soon I am entwined by the albino sheet boa constrictor. Waves of pain wash over me as I uncoil the sheets.

Neo wasn't any help. "Could be another terrible night, you know. It's surely starting out that way. Doesn't seem to be much you can do about it, huh? You know that each time you try to quiet down to rest, the pain just gets louder. I mean, I'm doing what I'm supposed to do, reminding you of the day's events and whatnot. But it just feels like you're not trying to fall asleep. You are failing at it, you know."

The "you're not good enough" button – grr! It always hits a tender spot, triggering a surge of anger mixed with worthlessness. Deep breaths as I let out a long sigh of exasperation. Over my life, this button has been pushed more times than our politicians have sent tweets.

Neo pauses for a moment before offering, "Lots of memories of pain are connected to punishment, oppression, and self-worth issues. But this is an old familiar path, and you know what happens if you take that fork in the journey."

Moving along this well-trodden path, I know I can tune out those "old voices." They offer nothing more than the cackling of old hens.

You can do this – breathe in 1, 2,3. Breathe out 1, 2,3.

Let go and allow.

Neo jumps in, "We're not finished here. There are a few things to worry about. You are trapped in a cycle of poor sleep – increased emotions – increased pain – poor sleep."

The logic of Neo's interruption, illustrated with an emotional soundtrack, started to send me into a worry spin like a dog chasing its tail. The more I worried, the more I became stuck in the worry. If I kept spinning, then I was going to cross over the "you will never get back to sleep" threshold. Need to return to the pause between.

You can do this – breathe in 1, 2,3,4. Breathe out 1, 2,3,4.

Let go and allow.

As the first glimmers of change appear in my conversation, Neo warns, "You know the pain is just going to get louder when you do this."

Very firmly, without anger, I say, "I know that I can move into a pause between and then to a mental quiet place. I've done it before, and I can do it again."

I can do this – breathe in 1, 2,3,4. Breathe out 1, 2,3,4.

Let go and allow.

Neo senses the changes. The perceptions of pain and discomfort are slowly lowering. The cool night breezes tuck me into a bed that suddenly feels very embracing. There is no need to talk about the pain.

Breathe in 1, 2,3,4. Breathe out 1, 2,3,4.

Let go and allow.

Breathe in 1, 2,3,4. Breathe out 1, 2,3,4.

Breathe in.

Breathe out.

Fifteen minutes later, I am sound asleep.

The Suntan Isn't Worth It

This essay starts with a short fictional story but is based on an experience shared to me by another couple dealing with PD.

Betty slapped George hard. No response. She dialed 911. PD had forced George into early retirement. He loved basking in the sun, diving into a good book, and working on his tan on the deck of their home.

Betty was in the kitchen when she saw him slumped over in the chair. This wasn't the first time George had responded so severely to the summer heat. Two other times, he had reacted to the heat in the same way. His heart rate was slower, almost imperceptible. His face was an ashen shade.

Waiting for the ambulance, Betty cradled George's face in her hands, and with tears streaming down her face commanded, "Don't you die on me." To herself, she said, "The suntan isn't worth it."

Like George, heat hits me hard. A small increase in air temperature above 75 degrees can have me prone for hours, if not the whole day. Relief isn't found by not moving or not engaging in any activity. I can have a difficult time in the shade or in the house if the temperature rises. I follow the recommendations to avoid heat stroke – I hydrate with water, I get any outside activities done in the earlier, cooler parts of the day, I wear light, loose clothing. We have a house cooled by central air. But despite all these precautions, I can sense the losing battle with the heat as it rises. A comfortable summer day for others becomes a debilitating challenge for me due to these heat attacks.

This reaction to heat is an attack on my ability to function, a magnified response, like my descriptions of fatigue and pain.

Researchers identify that heat intolerance is different than heat illnesses like heatstroke. It is usually a symptom of endocrine disorders, drugs, or other medical conditions, rather than the result of too much exercise or hot, humid weather. Up to 64% of PD patients report thermodysregulation, which includes symptoms of heat and cold intolerance as well as excessive sweating.[96]

PD patients have problems with their autonomic nervous system, which controls sweating. While perspiration helps regulate the body's temperature, too much or too little perspiration can result in overheating.[97]

Many of us are experiencing warmer temperatures for longer periods of time wherever we live. I used to be able to spend hours in the sun, get a tan, and enjoy being outside. Now I can't. Time for a tweak in the wellness map. I shift from thinking I can work in some heat to "it's not worth the suntan." It's not something to ignore or push through, distracting the mind away from the physical issues, hiding head in the sand. It must be met straight on with reason and sensible action. Most of us are not yogi masters who can change body temperatures at will. We must use what we know and take steps to prevent serious harm from happening. This is my strong voice telling me not to take this risk lightly. I tend to push myself too hard.

The symptoms of heat intolerance can vary from person to person, but may include:
- Body temperature that feels hot in moderately warm temperatures
- Excessive sweating or not sweating enough in the heat

---

[96] "Excessive Sweating in Parkinson Disease," by Neepa Patel, M.D., in *Michigan Parkinson's Foundation*, undated.

[97] LeDoux M.S. "Thermoregulatory Dysfunction in Parkinson's Disease." In Pfeiffer R.F., Bodis-Wollner I. (eds) *Parkinson's Disease and Nonmotor Dysfunction (Current Clinical Neurology)*. Humana Press, Totowa, NJ, 2013. https://doi.org/10.1007/978-1-60761-429-6_14

- Exhaustion and fatigue during warm weather
- Nausea, vomiting, or dizziness in response to heat
- Changes in mood when too hot

If you experience any of these symptoms, time to get out of the heat![98] It's just not worth the suntan.

Caressed by Calmness – So What?

Wow! That was intense. I was just sitting in the space between with no expectation beyond a quiet mind, just allowing the moment to bloom, when suddenly the moment transformed into this encompassing sense of being caressed by calmness. Even more surprising, the calm stayed with me for part of the day and it came with almost the absence of pain.

The experience was not that long – minutes, not hours – but long enough for me to recognize it as an extended well-being moment. During the daily routine of morning self-care and household chores, the memory of it stayed with me. I thought my PD had taken this from me. It's been many years since the last time I felt such radiant calmness.

It has been weeks since being caressed by calmness. Now I am muttering to myself, "Toss this essay in the trash. It's just not getting to the point." I was emotionally upset after a rough couple of weeks with multiple stressful events back-to-back. It would have been nicer to have had the option to revisit the calmness during these trying weeks. Nothing I tried led me back to those calm moments, and I asked myself, "You had this soothing experience – so what? What good is it if you can't get back there?"

The extended well-being moment has passed, leaving

[98] "Everything you need to know about heat intolerance" by Zawn Villines, medically reviewed by Elaine K. Luo, M.D. in *Medical News Today Newsletter*, May 21, 2019.

behind bits and pieces of memory that were fading with time. Just two weeks after the experience, trying to rekindle the memory found it lacking in the clarity and healing power of the original experience. Therein lies the problem. I couldn't easily return to revisit nor could I recreate it in memory, so what good was this experience? The benefit is found in understanding the possibility that the experience represents. Within that possibility are found the tweaks for my wellness map.

There are many benefits to regular meditative practice. A study reported in the Journal of the American Medical Association cites, "Mindfulness yoga appeared to be an effective and safe treatment option for patients with mild-to-moderate Parkinson disease for stress and symptom management; further investigation is warranted to establish its long-term effect and compliance."[99]

In mindfulness-based intervention (even without the yoga), participants in a 2015 study reported in *Parkinson's Disease* journal were asked to actively observe sensations in the body. The authors state, "Pain is a troublesome, frequently reported and complex, multifactorial nonmotor symptom in PD and the exact relationship between the disease and pain remains to be elucidated."[100] The results of their study indicate that mindfulness training may empower the individual to learn how to strengthen internal resources for coping with chronic disease, and restore some degree of self-determination in the experience of living with PD.

The calmness experience left me with a strong reminder

[99] Kwok, Jojo YY, et al. "Effects of Mindfulness Yoga vs Stretching and Resistance Training Exercises on Anxiety and Depression for People With Parkinson Disease: A Randomized Clinical Trial." *JAMA Neurol.* 2019;76(7):755-763. doi:10.1001/jamaneurol.2019.0534
[100] Pickut, Barbara, et al. "Mindfulness Training among Individuals with Parkinson's Disease: Neurobehavioral Effects." *Parkinson's disease* vol. 2015 (2015): 816404. doi:10.1155/2015/816404

of what is possible if I practice meditation more consistently. When I can meditate, the sensations of pain often start to rise, and at that point I need to enter the "pause between" and search for an alternative fork in the road. I do not want to be pulled into old habits. If I cannot sweep away the habitual patterns of thought and action, the calmness becomes more and more a distant memory. I must bring the event into play as part of my daily conscious thought.

The radiant calmness experience helped me by putting a clear and obvious road sign at the fork on my wellness map. The sign reads, "Calmness this way." This radiant calmness changed me by smoothing out the rough edges. It comes with tools useful against the weeds of unrest: patience, tolerance, and compassion.

Life's problems can be perceived as less burdened with emotion. The answer to the question, "So what happens if I let go?" is found in holding on to the possibility of change and then practicing moving in that direction every day. Every day has pain from PD. But it also provides the opportunity to practice calmness despite the discomfort.

I remain deeply moved by the reminder that at one time I lived closer to this radiant calmness.

Maybe at one time we all did.

Explaining, Not Complaining: Conversation with Neo

Pain visits me all the time now. There are multiple days with high levels that make me nauseated. I am sick and tired of having to say how sick and tired I feel. Experimenting with a new approach: responding to the pain in a dispassionate way, making observations, and providing explanations.

Neo (my neocortex who acts as my "alter ego" in brain

conversations) snickers, "Who are you kidding? You can't sit with five days of high pain without the Grouch showing up and leaving behind a trail of consequences." Neo tends to be a bit of a naysayer, much like Eeyore in the Winnie the Pooh books.

"Not true," I quickly retort. "The last two five-day stretches of bad pain, I did not let the Grouch speak in public. Mrs. Dr. C. shared her sincere gratitude on this accomplishment. It makes it easier on her, and in doing so, makes the home less stressful, decreasing my total pain level."

Neo replies, "I'm not talking about just zipping the lip. I'm talking about that inner dialog, the way you speak about the high levels of pain to yourself. What happened the other night after five days with high pain?"

I let out a deep sigh. "That was a difficult night, following a difficult week. It seemed like so many events were crashing around me. I tried to quiet my thoughts, but the pain was too loud, overpowering, and eventually all consuming."

Neo challenges my perception. "Did you see how you talked to yourself about this high pain experience?"

Reflecting back, I admit, "Yep. With every pain surge, I complained about how miserable I felt. There wasn't an external Grouch for others to see, but he showed up in my thoughts – a lot!"

"Exactly! I saw him lurking about," Neo exclaims. "It is the Grouch you have to change if you seek improved well-being. It's easy to complain, and you have plenty of company on social media. But finding a different path, implementing healthy solutions, that's where the hard work happens."

I've seen glimmers of a different inner dialog. Rather than reacting to the high pain, I should be sitting in the "pause between" and observing with as little emotion as possible. Analyze the pain and report back to Neo like a journalist covering a story. A new inner dialog needs to continue to keep the Grouch at bay. It's a dialog about being caressed with calmness, about knowing this is possible at any time, and making the calmness the focus of my attention.

"Nice idealism," Neo says, waving his brain neurons at me. "You know you haven't been fully successful at this yet."

I sigh, "True, I haven't achieved a perfect day. Maybe I never will. But I am trying every day to improve." Taking a deep breath to calm emptions stirred by Neo's pointing out my failings, I continue. "But I also find that seeking quietude within the 'pause between' helps me. I'm facing one day at a time while doing all I can to implement a new pattern of thought and behavior. It's just small incremental steps right now, but I'm happy with the progress."

With that Eeyore tone, Neo reminds me, "You know how hard this is to accomplish."

I stand, move to the windows, and look out on the perennial gardens. The summer colors are starting to diminish, but the plants have plenty of blooms still. "You know, Neo," I say calmly, "life is like gardening in many ways. One shovel full of dirt, plants placed in complementary shapes and colors, and a broad level path to walk, pause, and enjoy. Showing up and accomplishing those baby steps every day eventually brings forth a garden of wonder and delight."

Neo and I are quiet together while we walk the garden path.

We Just Want to Have Fun

"Fun" is one of those short "f-words" that doesn't have a strong history in our home. Mrs. Dr. C. and I are from the "nose to the grindstone, make it happen, pursue the American dream" generation. Oh, and try to live up to Gandhi's saying, "Become the change you wish to see in the world." We can be intense.

With all those noble ideals, we find that doing "fun" things is difficult for us. We don't know how people take "fun" vacations. We have never been successful at doing that. Sure, we want to have fun times in our retirement years, but with all the time commitments chronic illness demands, that little "f-word" requires more tweaks in the wellness map.

To illustrate how we just can't accomplish the standard idea of fun, I share this story about our attempts at a honeymoon. The first one, the one usually planned by newlyweds, never happened because my wallet was stolen at the wedding reception. So much for traveling without credit cards or identification. Four years later, we tried for a second honeymoon. During an idyllic trip to Maine, Mrs. Dr. C. developed a tremendous migraine – her first – so we cut the trip short. Twenty years later, we tried to combine a job relocation/house hunting expedition/vacation at my new jobsite in Reno with a stay at a casino. Heart-shaped velvet bed and all expenses paid by the company, but our minds were on finding a rental unit quickly and coordinating a 1,500-mile relocation with the movers. It was the last time we used a standard societal definition of fun as our own. Forty years later, we were more successful combining a trip to Arizona for a friend's wedding with exploring the countryside and downtown Phoenix. No other demands on our time except for dealing with chronic disease symptoms.

Changing behaviors so deeply ingrained in our lives is what tweaking the wellness map is all about, and it is never easy. We give ourselves permission to have "fun" and yet, at the same time, we must balance how to achieve said "fun." Used to be that we could be more spontaneous or at least show up for planned activities that have been on the calendar for weeks. Now, we tentatively agree to be somewhere, but roll with the day when it arrives.

We wake up each day knowing that each day must be faced as it presents. If there just isn't energy or physical ability to meet that obligation, we change the date and try to not feel guilty. It may seem strange to have to give ourselves permission to have fun, but we do this every day. If we listen only to that inner worker voice, then each day is just about the quest to accomplish something. "One more thing off the list!" Mrs. Dr. C. says, with as much glee as the Queen of Hearts in *Alice in Wonderland* chopping off heads.

But there is a new voice now. We still wake every day asking ourselves (and each other) "What are we going to accomplish today?" but it is tempered with knowing that each day must be evaluated on the morning of that day. Is this going to be a good day with enough energy to do what is on the schedule? We give ourselves permission to decline or reschedule activities based on how the day presents.

The new normal of traveling with chronic disease requires a separate medication bag, pillows and cover in the back seat of the car for those off periods, a cane for days where balance and coordination are a problem, scheduling the drive to allow a more leisurely pace, and a calendar that tries not to commit too many things in a week. We try to plan one meal at a restaurant while traveling to take a break from the drive, pull over more frequently at rest areas on the interstates, or make hotel accommodations for the night before to allow for rest to tackle the next day's commitment. More tweaking of the wellness map.

Perhaps we really do have fun. It just looks different than how other folks define it. Playtime and time experiencing a lightness of being are both part of fun and adjusting to PD, but so is creativity. Gardening, walking our forest path, genealogy, writing, reading, organizing our mineral collection, watching a movie, and just being together to share the journey[101] – we

---

[101] "Leisure, creativity and creative therapies." Published on European Parkinson's Disease Association (EPDA) website.

find our fun applying our talents to creative projects and shared moments together, and not letting PD and chronic disease ruin the day.

Defining a Sanctuary

"The mass of men lead lives of quiet desperation," wrote Henry David Thoreau while sitting on the edge of Walden Pond.[102] We live in a pandemic world, with income and political disparity threatening the pillars of well-being in democratic nations.[103] Kings of the oligarchy are viewed as pallbearers to the American dream.[104] Lost hope, anxiety, and absence of discernment fuel the flames of desperation. But exposure to the world need not mean becoming like the world. We can find peace in sanctuary.

A journalist and philosopher, Thoreau lived in a way that we would refer to now as "off the grid," self-sufficient in a cabin he built. He wanted to see if it was possible to break those chains of desperation by choosing to live a simple, less encumbered life. Thoreau pays homage to all the existential mystics and philosophers before him who found the true self only through the death of the ego. Letting go of old ways, habits, and old things is not easy. It helps the rebirth process

---

https://www.epda.eu.com/living-well/well-being/leisure-creativity-and-creative-therapies/

[102] Thoreau, Henry David. *Walden*, 1854.

[103] Wilkinson, Richard, and Pickett, Kate. *The Spirit Level: Why Greater Equality Makes Societies Stronger*. Bloomsbury Publishing; Revised, Updated ed. edition (May 3, 2011).

[104] "Baby Boomers Approach 65 – Glumly" by D'Vera Cohn and Paul Taylor, published on Pew Research Center Social and Demographic Trends, December 20, 2010.

if one can be enveloped and nurtured in a healthy sanctuary.[105]

Healing/sacred places are part of the human experience. These sanctuaries exist all over the world and are utilized by a wide diversity of cultures. Thoreau might disagree with me calling Walden Pond a sanctuary, but the reverence he held for the place and the support it provided him during his metaphysical journal fits my concept of a sanctuary.

Our home, after years of hard work, has transformed into our sanctuary. The beauty and sacredness of sanctuary can be created almost anywhere.[106] We think of it as a special place, or beauty and reverence where we find rejuvenation. Gradually, we eliminate the worldly toxins that always seem to creep into life, replacing them with beauty that inspires an internal shift toward well-being. We set aside time several times a to embrace our sanctuary. It has been worth the years of hard labor.

Sanctuary always has root in the natural world, like a garden or park[107] (the N in CHRONDI). But sanctuary is also framed within the mind, soul, and heart. Sanctuary is a holistic healing space that helps me with pain management, management of PD "off" periods, and decreases the negative effects of a bad day.

Most importantly, sanctuary is a safe place to let go of the stressors of life. One need not be an aesthetic – one who gives up worldly pleasures – to embrace well-being moments within a sanctuary. It is more about letting go of our attachments to things. It is the attachments which constrain our freedom to access the full benefits of sanctuary.

---

[105] Idler, Ellen. "The psychological and physical benefits of spiritual/religious practices." *Spirituality and Higher Education Newsletter,* vol. 4, issue 2, February 2008.

[106] Perriam, Geraldine. "Sacred spaces, healing places: therapeutic landscapes of spiritual significance." *The Journal of medical humanities* vol. 36,1 (2015): 19-33. doi:10.1007/s10912-014-9318-0

[107] https://sacredsites.com/

The question I ask myself is, "Would you walk away from all that you own in order to more fully understand that voice crying in the wilderness?" Twice in my life, I have done exactly that. Not an easy decision on my family, as there were moments of voluntary poverty. But it is not the poverty in and of itself which brings the radiance of sanctuary into view. It is the ability to totally let go.

In my research on advanced empathy, I describe a series of experiences that are common to both the healer (practitioner) and the patient (participant) when sharing a facilitated well-being moment. These are:

1) Agreement: the two reach a mutual agreement regarding the purpose of this special healing relationship.
2) Resistance: there is always resistance to sitting in a sacred space to experience well-being. This resistance can be explored if the sacred space is experienced as safe, and there is trust in the possibility of well-being as an outcome.
3) Letting go and catharsis.
4) Well-being is experienced.
5) Both participants undertake making meaning of the experience.

All five of these experiences are enhanced when both the participant and the practitioner surround and have embraced the sacredness of sanctuary. In the same way, our individual journey of wellness mapmaking is enhanced by sanctuary. It starts with an agreement on defining your personal sanctuary, your relationship to it, and how to use it.

Achieving a sanctuary is an important part of learning about shifting perspective. There are several essays on both topics because I feel it is such an important, and underutilized, therapy for people with PD. I hope the reader will explore this with me.

Embracing Sanctuary

The sunlight bounces its way through the swaying birches, projecting a shadow picture show on the lawn and garden shed. The light wind causes the fluttering leaves to sing in unison like waves on the shore. The family of hummingbirds – we have given them all names now – take turns showing off their aerial ballet at the feeder just feet from my rocking chair. The gardens are still blooming with cranberry-red coneflowers nestled between large-cupped orange and yellow daylilies. In the distance, I hear the sweet calming vibrato of our brook. It beckons me to embrace the support revealed within my sanctuary.

Sanctuary can be found, created, anywhere. It doesn't have to be Walden Pond or look like the description above. What is important is the frame of mind used when accessing sanctuary. Sanctuary is that place where the saying, "You get back out what you put in," really applies. If the awe and beauty of sanctuary are embraced while also experiencing the solitude, safety, serenity, and sacredness, then I know I am in the right frame of mind.

Sanctuary is more than a sacred physical place. The physical merely signals the senses to be ready for the well-being phenomena. The physical sanctuary supports the emotional and spiritual sanctuary. It is from this inner stance that I seek calm, and a trusting openness, and am ready to experience the journey. I have a relationship with my sanctuary and this "agreement" is the first step to incorporating sanctuary into a wellness plan.

Architects realize the importance of creating healthy living and work environments.[108] Designs for buildings and the

---

[108] "HOK and RSP Architecture Designing New Life Sciences and Innovation Research Center in Minnesota," published on Construction Forum, May 16, 2017.

areas they occupy, whether in a rural or urban setting, are incorporating a sense of sanctuary for well-being.[109] Providing for "green space," buffers, and integrating the natural environment are key concepts for architects. "Architecture helps shape the quality of our environments and can contribute to health and happiness," writes Karl Johnson.[110] Sanctuary is always rooted in the beauty of nature. The N in CHRONDI stands for Nature and its health benefits.

Let me share my story of sanctuary. The week had been terribly busy, more so than usual. It started with a trip to my general provider's office for fasting lab work. It's almost a two-hour drive to get there, and I was on an empty stomach until after the labs were drawn, which throws off my PD medications. The next day, there was the trip to Boston for VA services. That trip always takes two days, as we drive down the day before the appointment to break up the trip. We stay at a hotel and then get up the next morning to complete the four-hour drive and get to the appointment. The appointments are never fun. At least this one didn't require the providers to poke or prod or inject. Well, maybe some poking, but no injections.

Then we drove home, requiring another four hours on the road. With my rigid PD, every minute on the road becomes more uncomfortable. No time to rest because I'm back at the provider's office a day later for the lab results. The day after the doctor's appointment is errands and Mrs. Dr. C.'s hand-delivered application to the state offices for "designated caregiver" status. What we didn't have energy to do was attend was a live theater presentation on Galileo, celebrate our

[109] "Designing Wellness: What Influence Does Architecture Have on Health?" by Thomas McMullan, Opinion, published on Frieze, October 3, 2018.

[110] "Place and public health: the impact of architecture on well-being" by Karl Johnson, published in Health and Wellbeing, *The Guardian*, June 11, 2013.

anniversary, or go to the monthly get-together for New England Santa's Association. We make decisions every week about where to spend available free time, including letting go of some things in favor of time spent with sanctuary.

Weeks like the one I describe above are more difficult for me. I require several days to recuperate and recover. Days where the fatigue is almost overwhelming, and I can't return to my projects as much as I would like. My mind is tired, my body is drained, and my soul seeks out my sanctuary. I don't have to have faith that sanctuary will help. I know from personal experience that it will.

It may be your sanctuary can be created in your home: a favorite room, a comfortable chair. You can build a garden along a walkway. Perhaps you will find, as I do, that I can create several different areas, each unique to the landscape and plants and season. I enjoy the beauty of each special place within my quiet sanctuary. What is important is your ability to embrace that special sacred physical place, the sanctuary which offers you the greatest support for well-being.

Resisting Sanctuary: Conversation with Neo

BOOM! Abruptly out of bed, flashing lights reflecting on the bedroom walls disorient me. I sit on the edge of the bed and look out onto what should be morning sun, bringing to life the cherry red of bee balm against the backdrop of the white birches. But not today. Today, the sky is black. I thought it was night, but the clock says its morning. Rain hammers out a discordant melody on our metal roof. It's one of those gloomy, wet, cold days. It sure would be nice to curl up under the covers.

Neo shouts at a volume comparable to the thunder, "Heck, no! You have only two days until your big research

presentation."

I quickly snap back, "I know, I know." The cotton oasis beckons me to go fetal. Neo is quite annoyed with me.

"What are you thinking?" Neo inquires.

"Oh, nothing. You're right. I should look over the presentation, but I can't get motivated to do so. I'm so nervous that I can't even turn on my computer," I say in almost a whisper as I reach to pull the covers over me.

"Oh no, you don't. Get out of bed and let's face this fear. What's there to be afraid of? You know the material and you enjoy public speaking." Neo doesn't understand my concern with this latest development in my PD.

I retort, "It's not that at all. It's about my physical ability to do it. This summer, my PD symptoms got worse and there are times where I cannot perform motor tasks successfully. There is nothing I can do to stop these motor dysfunctions. What if one happens right when it is my turn to stand and give my presentation?"

"So, your fear of failure due to the possibility of motor freezing is preventing you from doing anything at all?" Neo replies with a slight sneer.

Somewhat defeated, I offer, "I could go back to bed."

Neo scoffs, "That's not going to solve anything. Why not enter your sanctuary for a while? You know that helps." Neo is pointing out what I already know, but it is not motivating me to act.

"Really?" I counter. "Look outside. It's not exactly walk-in-the-park conditions. Besides, my focus should be on how to make my presentation better." I move to the bathroom and start getting ready for the day.

Neo repeats, "Embracing sanctuary is not affected by the weather. Your senses and your mind can still take in all that sanctuary offers even in the rain."

I can feel my emotions starting to escalate. "I don't feel like calming down. I need the emotional energy to light up enough passion so I can break the chain of procrastination and the fears about my PD symptoms." I'm dressed and heading to the kitchen for breakfast.

Neo surveys my actions as I drop part of my breakfast on the floor. "You think you are more physically capable if you are all energized and full of passion?" Good thing Neo is above the physical and out of the way of any unintended physical harm.

"I..." pause and stare off to nowhere in particular. "I guess not. But it feels familiar and, in that way, safe. I can't quiet down enough to use sanctuary right now. Each time I move towards quieting, the pain gets so loud it's unbearable. That's certainly not conducive right now to getting my presentation ready." I am now pacing the floor as I continue to mutter about the presentation due in two days.

"Man, you are seriously stressed." Neo points out the obvious. He is adept at recognizing the situation is going downhill quickly. "Time in the sanctuary does help with stress. You know that stress unattended will just intensify all the PD symptoms – the physical, mental, emotional, and the psychological. Too many ripples in the pond with that big rock you're throwing at yourself."

Between mouthfuls of granola and orange juice, I say, "I'm sure. I don't have the time. Perhaps another day I could handle this. I can't look at that reflecting pond right now. I'm afraid that I will hate what I see."

"I know." Neo says. "The path is always here when you want to walk it and I'm with you too."

Neo and I watch the rain let up, leaving behind garden flowers painted with iridescent droplets reflecting off beams of sunlight poking through the storm clouds.

A Scientific Model of Sanctuary

Each time I seek sanctuary, there is resistance. I found a model of how sanctuary works and helps me to overcome that resistance.

I watched a lecture by professor Dr. Indre Viskontas, cognitive neuroscientist, in the television series *Brain Myths Exploded*.[111] She spoke about the brain as always having some level of background noise, and that conscious attention is given only to those stimuli which can break through that noise. It's a concept which matches with my conceptualization of the quiet mind as a mental state that is different from active conscious thought because the noise-to-signal ratio changes and use of threshold management changes. I just never painted my brain model that way before, but I really like the new colors.

Since hearing that lecture, the signal-to-noise ratio idea crawled its way through my web of interwoven knowledge on various types of attention and their application to chronic disease recovery. The practice of using sanctuary to promote well-being is linked to the practice of redirecting attention, including shifting perspective. PD affects brain areas that are responsible for moderating emotions and attention, dealing with stress, and overlearned motor sequences. I find I am less troubled by my chronic disease issues when sanctuary is in my life.

Here is a model of how I think sanctuary works. The first thing in the model is the foundation of a set of assumptions we agree to be true:

1) It's Alive: The brain generates electrical and chemical

[111] Indre Viskontas, Ph.D. *Brain Myths Exploded: Lessons from Neuroscience*. Available at https://www.thegreatcourses.com/courses/brain-myths-exploded-lessons-from-neuroscience.html

energy and is always "on" or "off." "Off" would imply brain death.

2) Brain Specialization: Certain areas of the brain are responsible for specific functions, such as motor memory, pain awareness, sensory input, and motor control.

3) Use it or Lose It: Use, or non-use, of the brain correlates with neural branching or neural snipping. More branches correlate with improved functioning of that brain area and communication to other brain areas. The more you use it, the easier it is to use. If you don't use it, then it's hard to overcome the resistance.

4) Consciousness is Attention to Signals Above the Noise: The brain is always processing neurochemical signals and creates a level of internal background noise, much of it subconscious, that acts as a filter, allowing us to attend to that which is deemed most important.

The signal-to-noise ratio filter is a fundamental part of both attention and memory and important to the model of sanctuary. In other words, one can get very easily overwhelmed. When the noise turns up, my ability to concentrate or process information goes down... way down. And PD just makes it harder to focus, tune in, and move forward.

On top of the model foundation is built the main body of the model – providing some understanding of how sanctuary works to promote lasting changes in well-being. I find that the following ideas help me move past the noise:

1) Conscious Perception is Not Fixed: The level at which signals exceed noise and become conscious perception is not a fixed boundary. We can be conscious of excessive stimuli and adapt to the demands of the situation. There are times when we are hyper alert and time seems to slow down (like being in a car skidding on icy roads). Consider what happens to conscious

perception when you fall asleep. Conscious perception level is not fixed.

2) Perception of "Noise" Can be Changed: The behavior of the "noise" can be altered through meditative practices. Instead of standing in a pond with raging waves of noise, we can be standing in still waters. Changing the way noise is heard changes the way life is perceived.

3) Threshold Tolerance Levels Can Be Changed: There is a signal threshold tolerance which, when exceeded, will result in dysregulated emotions. Meditative practices can increase threshold levels and unhealthy practices can lead to a lower threshold tolerance.

Now with the foundation up and the walls built, we can add the roof to our sanctuary model.

The last piece of the scientific model of sanctuary is the practice of early detection. It is using sanctuary to provide an early warning for us so we can avoid the consequences of dysregulated emotions. How many times have I said, or done, something in the heat of the moment only to regret it afterwards? We are creatures of desire and passion. Emotions are a language filled with rich information. The skill lies in being able to hear subtle emotion signals before they become a chaotic storm.

Developing an early warning system makes a huge impact on wellness. The sooner I can detect any abnormal increase in signal intensity pushing me over the top and possibly spinning out of control (at least in my head, if not my actions), the more likely it is that I can be successful in controlling the threshold. Sanctuary works because it supports my internal early detection system. This happens because attention, perspective, and possibility of change have been shifted. Shifting into the "pause between" is a new way of seeing old problems or old models. It all ties back to the science model of sanctuary.

For me, the three most important steps I can take to manage my chronic disease are: 1) Arrange the best medical team; 2) Attend to physical equilibriums: exercise, sleep, and eat well; and 3) Practice using sanctuary in combination with a wellness map.

Letting Go is Not Forever Gone

Letting go is a constant theme with PD. What used to be easy is now challenging. Gone are the days of hiking for miles or spending hours in the gardens digging, hauling, lifting. Gone are those endless days when 24 hours of project immersion got me through complex problem solving and four college diplomas. Can't do it the same way anymore. Letting go of these expectations on myself is not as easy and the process of letting go always presents itself at sanctuary's door. It is never totally gone.[112]

Judith Sills, Ph.D., states, "It's an axiom of psychology that we are some recombination of all of our yesterdays. To move forward wisely, we are therefore often urged to look back. But there's a point where appreciation and analysis of the past become gum on your psychological shoe. It sticks you in place, impedes forward motion, and, like gum, it doesn't just disappear on its own. You need to do some scraping."[113]

Ralph Waldo Emerson said, "A foolish inconsistency is the

---

[112] "Important Tips on How to Let Go and Free Yourself," Ilene Strauss Cohen, Ph.D., published on *Psychology Today*, August 7, 2017.
See also: "Letting Go: What should medicine do when it can't save your life," Atul Gawande, Annals of Medicine, published on *The New Yorker*, August 2, 2010.
[113] "Let It Go!", Judith Sills Ph.D., published on Psychology Today on November 4, 2014.

hobgoblin of little minds."[114] When you can't let go, you are haunted by the hobgoblin. You can't let go and have nothing to replace it because the hobgoblin will rush back to fill the void. Sanctuary holds safety and sacredness in place of the void, allowing the possibility of well-being to unfold.

Letting go is learning to live with the bad things that happen. Not by eradicating memory, but by shifting attention and perception. In my quest to let go and accommodate chronic PD symptoms, I turn to sanctuary. I know I am using sanctuary appropriately because I run smack into resistance. It is hard to let go of old habits, old scars, and old voices playing on old tapes. Letting go is full of detours and wrong turns. I'm always learning more about how to let go. It is always a process – never done.

John M. Grohol, Psy.D., on the website psychcentral.com[115] identifies some key elements to the "letting go" process:

1) Make the decision to let it go. Making the conscious decision to let it go also means accepting you have a *choice* to let it go.

2) Express your pain – and your responsibility.

3) Stop being the victim.

4) Focus on the present – the here and now – and joy.

Tony Robbins adds, "Many of us get stuck in the past because of our need for certainty. We all need to feel certain that we can avoid pain and, ideally, find some comfort in our lives. By identifying your emotional habits, you can start to make the shift toward actively conditioning yourself toward a more positive experience. You can learn how to let go of the past in a way that makes you feel lighter and freer instead of

---

[114] Emerson, Ralph Waldo. *Essays, First Series*, published on American Transcendentalism Web.

[115] "Learning to Let Go of Past Hurts: 5 Ways to Move On," John M. Grohol, Psy.D., published on Psych Central, July 30, 2018.

fearful."[116]

Through most of our lives, so much of our self-identity is defined by what we do (rather than who we are). Strip away the things that we used to be able to do, and we feel like a naked person without the clothes we used to wear that defined us. PD can strip that identity.

So often social conversation turns to "What do you do for a living?" and I want to reply, "I'm just trying to survive." But I don't. I say I'm a writer. People who still see me as the person I used to be, or people that say, "But you look so good, how can you feel sick?" can't see the struggle of letting go that drains my energy and creates overwhelming fatigue.

"Those who mind don't matter and those who matter don't mind."[117] Family, friends, and some medical providers often do not fully understand how letting go carves away the substance of identity whittling it down to a splinter. More loss thrown on a plate already overflowing with dead bones.

For me, letting go occurs on many levels – sensations, emotions, thoughts, and pain. Sanctuary is not just a place to "feel good." Sanctuary gives me the strength and calmness to

---

[116] "How to let go of the past to release the past: You must focus on your present and future," Robbins Research International, published on TonyRobbins.com, undated.

[117] "Those who matter don't mind, and those who mind don't matter" was FDR presidential advisor Bernard Baruch's often-quoted response to Igor Cassini (a popular society columnist for the New York Journal American) when asked how he handled the seating arrangements for all those who attended his dinner parties. The quote first appeared in *Shake Well Before Using: A New Collection of Impressions and Anecdotes Mostly Humorous* (1948) by Bennett Cerf, p. 249. The full response was "I never bother about that. Those who matter don't mind, and those who mind don't matter." This anecdote has also become part of a larger expression, which has been commonly [and incorrectly] attributed to Dr. Seuss, even in print, but without citation of a specific work: "Be who you are and say what you feel, because those who mind don't matter and those who matter don't mind."

face my demons, mourn losses, and at the same time move forward into the future, and find peace with myself and with those around me. Letting go is not totally losing memories even when interwoven with the hard times. Letting go is not forever gone. It remains at sanctuary's door, opening the possibility of well-being.

Looking back grants me a fresh look at the process of letting go. It is not something I could comprehend fully until I went through it and could benefit from hindsight. It does get better if I stay true to the quest of living better with a chronic disease. Acceptance for me is tied to a deeper understanding of the disease and what I can and cannot change.

Making Sense of It All

Wellness map in hand, I pass through the fog of conflict that is my life and agree to enter sanctuary. Letting go of resistance, I surrender myself to the well-being and bliss experience. Caressed by calmness, the fog has lifted. Like a crisp fall day, the colors are vibrant and the view breathtaking. In the distance is something not seen before. This is the destination I must strive toward.

It beckons to me, constantly whispering in my ear, "come to me and discover what you need." It's all making sense to me, now.

Our brains are wired to make connections. Not just neural ones, but associative ones. When we have a new experience, we associate that experience with other similar experience memories. The farther the new experience is from the known, the more difficult it is to do this association.

Well-being and bliss moments can be so different from our history of experiences that the effort to connect associations is difficult; so difficult that procrastination often follows. "I can't make sense of this, so I'm not going to do anything about it until I can." It's a cautious approach I've taken many times in my life. Eventually, I get splinters from sitting on the fence too long.

"The unexamined life is not worth living," is a famous dictum by Socrates as described in *Plato's Apology*. Epicurus' philosophy on happiness is composed of three things: good companionship, being self-sufficient and free from everyday life and politics, and making time and space to think things through. Epicurus would advise not to spend money as temporary relief for a bad day, but rather take time out and reflect and contemplate. Socrates, on the other hand, has a different stance. Socrates believed you should review and examine every aspect of your life so you can get the best out of it. A life bereft of meaning and purpose lacks action guided by that purpose. Meaning and purpose are part of a healthy self-concept.

Making sense of well-being moments can be challenging because they are often scarce, and we have little experience in doing so. Well-being moments always come with useful information. Without that, they are just superficial, fleeting, "feel good" moments. Taking that information and turning it into wisdom for a lifetime requires wrestling with it, using it, and integrating it into life – use it or lose it. It often helps to have an experienced guide. Teachers of the mystic traditions suggest mentoring in a sanctuary is one way to assist in the meaning-making process.

How we make sense of everything is vital to our movement forward, against the challenges, the setbacks, the frailty that we encounter. Making sense of it gives us meaning and purpose throughout our journey with PD and through the rest of our lives.

Procrastination and Other Demons

It was one of those ugly days. PD symptoms were maxing out. I couldn't breathe with the viral infection I picked up. Mrs. Dr. C. was out of the house with an appointment, no shoulder to lean on. I was totally lacking in motivation to do anything that required more thought than needed to boil an egg. And... today was my deadline day to write the next column.

Feeling like I can't write the column and being unable to write are two quite different things. Sorting out the hesitation to engage in motor action from apathy and what looks like procrastination is complex with PD because of the various causes of failing to initiate motor action. Like most PD symptoms, there is not a "one size fits all," but for me, just taking the time to sort out the differences helps me to avoid the cyclic trap of responding to feeling like I can't engage. I work on this every day. Because of this and because I always try to show up where I need to be, people will comment on how good I look with PD.

"You are an inspiration to us all," was given as a compliment. I nodded and smiled, not knowing how to respond. There is a certain level of presentation that I take to avoid demonstrating my disabilities. Perhaps it is selfish, but I think trying to present as a "normal" social being is important when I interact with other people. It can be difficult at times when my irritability is at its peak, my stumbling and dropping things are so clearly evident. I'm constantly self-monitoring to avoid embarrassing or uncomfortable situations where someone might not see beyond the PD to the person I still think I am. I look at my life and see those things that I try to do to the best of my ability. It takes a lot of effort (both physical and mental), and sometimes what I want to do is difficult to achieve. Thomas Edison said, "success is 10% inspiration and 90% perspiration."

Procrastination and its root causes prevent people from turning vision into actuality. The wellness map lays folded on my dresser and sanctuary lies just beyond the curtains drawn tight. There are days when I just don't have the energy for them. It's not procrastination. Fatigue and pain add to an ugly day, making it difficult to accomplish tasks. But I work on letting go of the voice that says, "You're a bad person because you are not getting things done," replenishing my thoughts with the much calmer "Let it go, you will have better days" voice.

I also have lucid moments, and these are precious to me. I give myself permission to treat the difficult disease days with as much reverence as I give to the good moments. I also know that my wellness map used with sanctuary will decrease the number of bad days and increase the frequency of lucid moments. It opens the possibility for well-being moments.

I know all this. I know I should get off the sofa and engage, but there are times where I just can't. I'd rather put it off until tomorrow and do something different, usually tied to more immediate gratification. This is procrastination. It can easily become a habit as easily indulged as eating chocolate or ice cream or surfing through cable television. Too many inspirations get taken away because we embrace procrastination.

There are plenty of reasons given for putting off today what we can do tomorrow:

"It's too hard."

"My emotions are blocking progress."

"I want to avoid the pain of doing this – whether physical pain or mental fear of failure."

"I need comfort, not risks."

The most common cause is a somnolence of mind induced by procrastination. Finding the passion, the calling, purpose, and meaning to act are thoughtful actions. These are patterns incompatible with procrastination. It has been my observation that those who procrastinate are filled with ideas of how the world should be and yet leave the fire in the belly without fuel. Maybe next time someone will say, "You're a perspiration to us all."

A Pat on the Back: Conversation with Neo

"Wow! Your 50th column. You should feel proud," exclaimed Neo over our shared breakfast ruminations.

"Not really," I reply without hesitation. "I feel humbled and in awe. I have been writing about these topics for decades. To be given the honor of a column is a blessing. I am hopeful that I touch on issues that other people face."

Neo pushes a little bit. "Don't you think you deserve a pat on the back for all that hard work?"

The concept of ego gratification pushes my emotional buttons. "A pat for what? I am just following a calling and showing up well prepared. There's no need for an ego massage."

"That's not what I mean," Neo snaps back. "Comments from readers said the columns were very professionally written, they helped them feel better dealing with their medical issues, and they look forward to reading them each week."

Calmly I reply, "I am so incredibly grateful for my readership, but their praise doesn't dictate the writing. I can't write to seek acclaim if the writing is to remain authentic from my life experiences."

"So, you are just going to let this 50th column pass by without a pat on the back?" Neo says tersely.

To Neo, getting recognition for something has been important since childhood. Seeking recognition or receiving praise has been a long-standing desire, almost habitual, and I know it to be a slippery slope. Facing and working through medical challenges or working to establish a means of communication for fellow sufferers with PD doesn't fit well with such ego-driven goals.

Between sips of my morning juice, I counter, "It's not about me. Never has been and never should be. It's about the message. It's about crafting the best voice for sharing that message of hope with all who wish to read it. Ego will only get in the way."

Neo gazes out the window and sighs. "So, you are going to do nothing then? Maybe you just don't feel worthy."

I reply, "My worthiness is my own business and not subject to a culturally shaming guilt trip. There is no entitlement, no guarantees. This life owes me nothing. I don't write for expectations of rewards. The accolades, like fame, are illusory. Illusions cannot provide a sound foundation for authentic writing."

Neo, frustrated by my response, says, "I don't get it. It's normal to feel proud. It's the 50th column written by you!"

With a pat, I comfort Neo, "Normal has never been anything but a bell curve point for me. There is no measure of normality that can direct excellence or increased well-being. Pride is normal and it is ego-driven, not message-driven. Pride is defensive, superficial, quick to judge, and so often built on a crumbling foundation of ignorance. It can't direct my actions or thoughts."

Neo responds, "I'm saying it's OK to acknowledge your efforts. That isn't false pride. I'm saying it's OK to show a little self-kindness. You deal with a lot of issues in your life – much of it medical or related to how you deal with symptoms, accessing medical care, progression of the disease, and family and friends who don't always understand what is going on or can't show the level of support you might need at the moment. They don't see how difficult it is to wake up every morning and try to keep going despite the setbacks and difficulties.

What they see is the result of all that effort. They think they see how good you look and not what it takes every day to travel the path."

Neo is right in that aspect. I can be too hard on myself sometimes. If there's one thing I'm proud of, it would be my persistence in continually showing up well prepared – day after day, year after year. For those days where PD or my vision cause my life to be upended or adjusted on a moment's notice, then I work through it the best that I can and hope for the next day to be just a little bit better. If I can share any measure of hope through my experiences, or a sense of a shared community, then that is the best reward I can ever receive.

Neo agrees. "Yeah! That deserves a pat on the back."

The Ruin of a Sedentary Life

Wailing, with tears flowing, I cry out, "I feel terrible! I can't even think straight!" Mrs. Dr. C. runs over and hugs me hard. I am lost and with nothing left to give.

This is one way "crossing the threshold" affects my life. It happens. It's the result of things piling on things, the old ways of coping not working, and stress pushing me over the edge. All starting with the ruin of a sedentary life.

It was an ongoing disaster. I injured muscles overdoing in the garden. With rigid Parkinson's, it is the worst thing to put my muscles into further spasms and rigidity.[118] Recovery time

---

[118] Cano-de-la-Cuerda, Roberto, PT; Pérez-de-Heredia, Marta, OT; Miangolarra-Page, Juan Carlos, MD, PhD; Muñoz-Hellín, Elena, PT; Fernández-de-las-Peñas, Cesar, PT, PhD. "Is There Muscular Weakness in Parkinson's Disease?," *American Journal of Physical Medicine & Rehabilitation*: January 2010 - Volume 89 - Issue 1 - p 70-76 doi: 10.1097/PHM.0b013e3181a9ed9b

was weeks, which led to too much time on the computer. The eye disease and vision loss sustained earlier in the spring still had not compensated, so I had an increase in vertigo and migraines. Medication adjustment led to further nausea and a trial on "natural" medication led to an allergic reaction. With all of this, I had loss of appetite leading to losing more weight than I should have. Was it over? Not quite; I had exposure to a particularly nasty virus that really hit hard. With no exercise, extremely poor sleep, and all the above, it was the ruin of this writer's sedentary life.

I know that this situation is not good for me. At the same time, and in contradiction, there is also resistance to moving out of the situation. Easier to do things as they have been done in the past than to change. Even though I knew the old coping skills, like heavy exercise and gaming, were much easier before the PD, they are just not as effective now. There was procrastination. There were things I knew I should have done but didn't. I am not ruling out ignorance as a cause. There were many things about muscle injury recovery that I thought I knew, but afterwards came to know more. The amount of stress I was putting myself through to meet what I perceived as important demands on my life and time was unhealthy. The cruel fact of it all was that I could no longer recover from muscle injury in the way that I used to. I had to adapt to a new way to heal.

I can't find much scientific research on rigid Parkinson's[119] and the effect of hard exercise or recovery from muscle injury. More education is needed to help those who are trying to maintain an exercise regimen. To help, I created Exercise with Parkinson's Information Page (www.DrC.Life) with a list of Internet sources.

I realize also that my inattention to the changes I'm

---

[119] "Symptoms – Rigidity." By Editorial Team, published on Parkinson's Disease.net, February 28, 2017.

undergoing can place additional burdens on people around me. I am trying to learn to change my actions and not be irritated for failing to remember what I cannot do these days. So, my internal dialog is working on "out with the old and in with the new me." These are my well-being mantras:

1) If I can't do it like I did before, then I need to put the time in to learn a new way.

2) Vary my exercise regimen; adjust for recovery from injuries and the off periods.

3) Remember to warm up, stretch, and prepare for any planned hard exercise.

4) Keep hydrated. Use the belt attachment to carry my water bottle so I don't lose it or forget where it is.

5) Take the time to recover from anything strenuous. It used to take a day; now it can be two or three days.

6) Think about proper mechanics when doing tasks. I must figure out another way to cut down and move trees!

The ruin of a sedentary life was the result of many actions which exacerbated the muscle injury problem rather than adding to healing. Old ways, old talk, don't work anymore. Because the muscle rigidity and weakness has jumped another plateau in the chronic disease progression, I must teach myself a new way to exercise.[120] It can't be business as usual, because doing the usual just isn't working well anymore.

Now is the time to put the new wellness map into play – every day, with a healthy dose of self-kindness.

---

[120] "12 Types of Exercise Suitable for Parkinson's Disease Patients." Wendy Henderson in Social Clips, published on Parkinson's News Today, July 31, 2017.

Don't Worry, Be Happy

Not taking anything away from *Mad* magazine's Alfred E. Newman or singer-songwriter Bobby McFerrin, but the idea that a pair of rose-colored "don't worry, be happy" glasses will change my life for the better never sat well with me. Pollyanna is not a guest in my home.

"Look at all the wonderful things in your life. All your needs are provided for – no worries," someone said to us recently as we described the temporary ruin of stagnation. But for me, pouring saccharin sentiments over the burnt toast of my life won't remove the blackened flavor.

I write often about having a positive, action-based wellness plan. But it's an "A + B = C" approach: Attitude and behavior equal consequences. The positive outlook is wisdom based and compassion engaged. It is not based on my looking at the glass half full. One can try to view the chronic disease glass as being half full, but for me the reality is that it is also half empty at the same time. This is not to say I don't wish that the muscle and other PD symptoms were not there. It's just not an action plan – more of a "I'm tired of this right now" statement.

Many authors have extolled positive thinking: Norman Vincent Peale, Norman Cousins, among others. Choosing how to act, think, and feel creates patterns. We return to those patterns when times get tough. Or, as one person said, "fake it until you make it." It seems vacuous to assume that "faking" happiness will remove the causes of the unhappiness, or at the very least, make things appear better than they are. Well-meaning people who propose the "don't worry, be happy" solution do not have a clear understanding of what PD and other chronic diseases mean in coping with our daily lives. What is needed is a well-designed, and enacted, wellness map – not rose-colored glasses.

Although Mrs. Dr. C. and I have moments of frustration and utter despair, we manage to pull ourselves up once again – as we have throughout our lives – and find the inner and spiritual strength to continue. That is a lifelong habit for the two of us and we find that as a team, we can support each other through the continued challenges, taking turns with compassion and strength when the other one falters and feels the weight of the burden.

Do we worry? Yes, but gradually we move toward more acceptance. Are we happy? The glass remains half full and we are grateful for the happiness and blessings in our lives. But now it is time to replenish the glass and move into deeper compassion, and find strength in the belief that all things happen for a reason and in their own time. We will not shy away from the work that needs to be done in our lives and for others with chronic diseases.

Some people took this column to mean that one shouldn't try to cultivate a positive attitude. It is meant to address the habits of escaping the reality that the disease presents by creating a delusion of happiness. I cannot ascribe to the idea that avoiding an issue will cause the issue to disappear. The delusion can be harmful because it prevents one from clearly seeing the disease and then tackling it honestly with courage. Sometimes life just doesn't turn out the way we would hope. The reality is to create strength and courage in the face of adversity.

Relationship as Sanctuary

The healing relationship is a special relationship which holds a sacred place for people while they search for a path to experiencing well-being moments. This relationship offers every possibility for allowing that moment to occur. The healing relationship is a safe place, a sanctuary, which aims to facilitate the experience of well-being and then bear witness to that experience.

The healing relationship starts with an agreement to enter the compassion space for the purpose of exploring well-being. Some people enter the compassion space almost effortlessly without a great deal of resistance. Some can move to experience well-being in the compassion space quickly, while others take longer. Understanding how to sit with resistance and eventually let go is part of the relationship as sanctuary.

Resistance can be more intense with a relationship sanctuary than with sanctuary formed in connection to a place. There is the "other" person who may be difficult to reach out to or communicate deep personal feelings to. There are complicated interactions with family members in relationships of child, parent, sibling, or through marriage. We carry into each relationship interaction so many of the deep emotions that are tied to the memories of our relationships, good and bad. We enter the healing relationship with a "relationship stance" built upon our relationship history, and within that stance is resistance to sanctuary.

Working with a healer or guide as a form of relationship sanctuary can be immensely helpful. An experienced guide can help you see your resistance obstacles, help you to learn how to move around them, and then to experience a well-being moment.

Finding healing relationships while battling a chronic illness is tough, but necessary. We are by nature social creatures, and our health benefits from growth-nurturing relationships. I long for quality time with people where conversation explores the sacredness of life, not the sickness of strife. There are times when I want to talk about all the aches and pains. That's a natural course, and I seek out others' understanding or acknowledgement of what I'm going through. There are times where I do not. Chronic illness consumes much of my time, but it does not define me. I'll always have time for stimulating discourse on topics other than PD. My interest in the lives of others gives me pleasure in being able to share what they experience. It's not all about "me."

Everything seems so rushed these days. Thoreau said there was no need for people to travel so fast on those 25 mph locomotives. I chuckled, and then thought about how we are going even faster now. Relationships now are affected by a technological train that steamrolls into our lives without conscious consent. Texts and tweets, sometimes replacing even the obligatory holiday visits, give us brief glimpses of those we love as they go dashing about their lives.

I don't dash any more. Well, maybe to that emergency bathroom call, but not much else. I remember when I used to dash, both mentally and physically. Now I just can't push hard like that anymore. Too much stress, and with the progression of symptoms I experienced following the ruin of stagnation, life hit me hard. This summer my diseases took a turn for the worse, not a big crash off the road into a tree turn, but a noticeable bump in the road. The ruin of stagnation was part of the progression and everything is more difficult now than it was three months ago. It's hard to share all of this in a way that doesn't come across as a pity party. The relationship as sanctuary is a compassion space held for me to be heard, understood, not judged, welcomed, and embraced. In many ways, Mrs. Dr. C. does this day in and day without complaint. I get tired of being with myself more often than that.

Relationship as sanctuary has been my life's work, and I find the more I learn, the less I seem to know. OK, old saying, but it is so deeply poignant when applied to the sacred quality that can exist within the healing relationship. It is the best thing that I do as a human being in my service to humanity. Keep learning, keep reaching out and giving back.

Parkinson's Progression

Every day following the ruin of stagnation, it seems I have progressed from early Parkinson's to moderate Parkinson's. But I can't be sure. So many other things – like stress, injuries, medication changes, and getting older – could all be making it look and feel worse, and not have anything to do with the disease progression. To appease my quandary, I dove into the Internet searching for elucidation about PD progression.

We watched as Michael J. Fox and Muhammed Ali were changed by the disease. Granted, their Parkinson's symptoms were dramatic. Their body movements gradually became less fluid; tremors were very pronounced. Over time, the movement challenges became more noticeable – a progression. The common lexicon in the PD community is to use the terms "early," "middle," and "late stage" PD to describe this progression. It mostly makes sense and matches what providers identify with PD patients. But it doesn't help me in my search of well-being possibilities.

Progression for me is more than "early," "middle," or "late." The disease will cause changes in me and my life. I accept that. It would be helpful for my wellness map if some of the pitfalls could be marked "danger ahead!" or "here's a list of supplies" to help me get past the hard parts of the chronic disease journey. Being well prepared is a strong part of wellness success. The progression of PD is not about stages (except very generally). It means having some idea about what can be done to slow the progression, or failing to do so, and how to know if progression is happening. Helpful knowledge about progression will be information which guides us and our families through what is sometimes a tortuous journey. It might make the trip easier.

Chatting with the PD community about progression reveals the deep-rooted idea that progression is unique to everyone. It would be useful if our understanding of progression could provide for each patient more details than, "It's unique to everyone and you will know when you get there." What's holding up the progress of understanding PD progression? Medical professionals determine PD progression through a brief office exam, patient report, and sometimes a standardized measurement tool or questionnaire. This is the system for collecting information about progression. It seems that PD can manifest itself in so many ways that providers often miss parameters or don't have the time to identify all of them. One symptom may be seeming to escalate while another is quiescent. Sometimes, it seems that a symptom may fail to materialize during the office exam (for instance, gait imbalance) but upon returning home, I find myself tripping and wobbling. That system fails when all people can say about progression is, "You'll know it when you get there." We need better information from early PD stages to understand progression from early to middle and beyond. However, using data from the existing data collection system, it is nearly impossible to do so, and so people are left without a clear understanding of what progression means to them.

An article[121] by Jorik Nonnekes, et. al., discusses the merits of the retropulsion test with the three most common methods: "(1) the pull test as described in the MDS-UPDRS scale; (2) using an unexpected shoulder pull, without prior warning; and (3) the push-and-release test." Although the validity of the tests is given a high degree of identifying progression of Parkinson's by providers, the authors of the article state that "the outcome can vary considerably due to variability in test execution and interpretation." The authors pose the explanation that falling results from the complex interplay

---

[121] Nonnekes, Jorik, et al. "The Retropulsion Test: A Good Evaluation of Postural Instability in Parkinson's Disease?," *Journal of Parkinson's Disease*, vol. 5, no. 1, pp. 43-47, 2015.

between gait, balance, cognitive decline, and environmental factors, and the retropulsion test captures only part of that. They conclude that "irrespective of its method of execution, the shoulder pull fails to predict future falls in PD." This is one example of the difficulty in using office visit data to predict future disease problems, like falling. So, while I "pass" the retropulsion test in the office (scheduled about an hour after my medications), at home in my "off period" I catch my foot drag on the floor, wobble from side to side, and just barely right myself and catch the fall before it happens.

It is difficult to see the early symptoms in a short office visit once every three to six months. Increasing the speed of care by shortening the in-office visit time has done nothing to improve health care for this ailing writer. It limits getting to know the patient better and increases the chance of being categorized as "that patient with PD." The provider can't see all the effects of the chronic disease even with a longer visit. We have good days and bad days, on and off periods, and life circumstances, all which make data collection on PD progression from that one 15-minute office visit problematic. It makes sense that early diagnosis and proper treatment should make a difference in progression. As far as I can tell, there are no good longitudinal studies that describe variation in progression because of treatment, of lack thereof. This applies even to exercise, my favorite Parkinson's treatment to slow down the progression,[122] and the effects of stress as my "most need to avoid" situation to prevent speeding up the progression.[123]

In additional essays on progression, I will offer a possible

---

[122] Lauzé, Martine, et al. "The Effects of Physical Activity in Parkinson's Disease: A Review." *Journal of Parkinson's disease* vol. 6,4 (2016): 685-698. doi:10.3233/JPD-160790

[123] Hiller, Amie, Joseph Quinn, and Peter Schmidt. "Does Psychological Stress Affect the Progression of Parkinson's Disease" (N5.002). Neurology Apr 2017, 88 (16 Supplement) N5.002

solution to the PD progression research problem. Maybe it will help to gather better information so we can make better choices that open well-being possibilities with PD.

Technology to Record Progression

The best we can say to patients about PD progression is "it's a process unique to each person" and there is a general change from early, to middle, and then to late-stage symptoms. This view of PD progression may be an artifact of limited data rather than a description of PD progression. We need new ways to measure PD symptoms as they change over time. We have the technology to create new devices that people can use over an extended period, across multiple settings and severity of "off periods."

I see progression as a change in the intensity and duration of both off periods and "bad" days. Although there are many longitudinal studies (for example, one on exercise[124]), it is hard to find any that measure changes in functioning in response to treatment during these difficult PD times. The devices proposed here might change that.

Better measurement of PD progression begins with a few assumptions. First, subtle early motion movement signs will appear prior to the more obvious symptoms, such as tremors or bradykinesia. Second, these early motor symptoms will be inconsistent and episodic. Third, we have the technology to build mobile monitoring devices.

I recently read that a patient being evaluated for reporting

---

[124] Miller, Stephanie A., et al. "Rate of Progression in Activity and Participation Outcomes in Exercisers with Parkinson's Disease: A Five-Year Prospective Longitudinal Study," *Parkinson's Disease*, vol. 2019, Article ID 5679187, 9 pages, 2019. https://doi.org/10.1155/2019/5679187

"internal tremors" showed no tremor sign on physical examination of his bare feet.[125] However, once he put his socks and boots on, an astute clinician noted that the left bootlace demonstrated a swinging motion, that when measured, fit the PD pattern of tremor. The patient didn't exhibit tremor with visual examination of his bare feet, but the shoelace reflected the underlying tremor!

A shoelace is not going to be a reliable measuring device, but it points out that slight motor changes exist that are difficult to detect. I've thought about two possible motor symptom detection devices that could be developed: a mobile swing monitor (MSM) and a fine motor skills test (FST). Both devices would be used in daily life, over the span of 10 days or so, to record and monitor movement fluctuation over time and across settings. Both use special sensors to track and record movement through three dimensions. The MSM, mobile sway monitor, uses five "movement in 3D space" sensors – one on each wrist, one on each ankle, and one on the belt – worn with recording hardware for all five sensors.

This is similar in appearance to wearable training weights.[126] These 3D movement monitors are the same used by Olympic and World Cup judges evaluating Shaun White's amazing snowboard flips and twists. They can be calibrated to measure the slightest variations in body movement. Worn over the span of several days, like a Holter monitor, the device would map the sway of the arms, legs, and body over time and across settings.

---

[125] Bloem, Bastiaan R., et al. "The Shaking Shoelace." *Journal of Parkinson's Disease*, 9:1, 249–250, 2019 (DOI 10.3233/JPD-181541).
[126] Takei, Yusuke et al. "Wearable muscle training and monitoring device." In *2018 IEEE Micro Electro Mechanical Systems (MEMS)*, pp. 55-58. IEEE, 2018.

FST: Fine Motor Skills Test

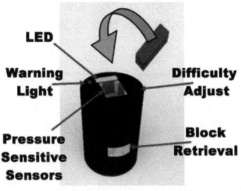

LED

Warning Light

Difficulty Adjust

Pressure Sensitive Sensors

Block Retrieval

Graphic by Dr. C. 2019

The FST also has a 3D monitor in a "soda can" receptor where the block is inserted. The FST will measure how the person adjusts position and control during fine motor skills, using the 3D monitor and four independent pressure-sensitive plates that record when the block is aligned or misses the attempt to insert the block into the hole. The plates can be positioned at different widths, using an adjustable difficulty setting, making it harder to fit the block in without touching the plates. The warning light goes off when the sensor plate is touched. The design concept is like that game of "Operation" where the person must remove toy "surgical" objects from the "anatomical" openings in the game "patient" without setting off the buzzer.

The data available from these two devices may be able to give PD patients and their providers more accurate clinical data about PD motion, tremors, and fine motor skills over a greater span of time. It could demonstrate in greater detail the progression of intensity and duration of both off periods and "bad" days. The data from these devices could serve as the beginning of a database on PD progression. If these devices are already being tested in the home with PD patients, then please sign me up!

Maybe readers can do what Mrs. Dr. C. has done. She took photos of the eggs I tried to crack into the dish for French toast. I tried twice. Both times, eggs on the counter and not in the bowl!

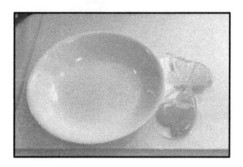

There is much excitement about using technology to provide outcome measures (TOMs) but, as we patients know, the technology is not being utilized in offices, with patients, to help understand the progression of PD.[127] Hopefully, that will change. In the meantime, I'll just ask my wife to crack the eggs for me.

From Zero to Sixty in Four Months: Conversation with Neo

Boom! A shot of sound that shakes the windows of the house. No, it's not interplanetary aliens with laser guns showing up in rural New England. It's just winter. We have a steel roof. When the temperature is exactly right, the snow

---

[127] Artusi, Carlo Alberto, et.al., "Integration of technology-based outcome measures in clinical trials of Parkinson and other neurodegenerative diseases." *Parkinsonism and Related Disorders*, Volume 46, Supplement 1, January 2018, Pages S53-S56. Published: July 26, 2017 DOI:https://doi.org/10.1016/j.parkreldis.2017.07.022 https://www.prd-journal.com/article/S1353-8020(17)30269-9/fulltext

slides off the roof with the force of a cannonball and impacts the ground and ice with just as much noise. Every winter, I've been out helping clear the snow. But not this year. The ruin of stagnation has forced me into nearly zero physical activity while I healed. Slow progress was made as I increased exercise each day from zero minutes to sixty minutes. It is awfully slow healing. I am not used to the slow pace and that nags at me, like a child wanting to get to the next carnival ride.

Neo interrupts my lament. "Well, it's been four months. What have you accomplished over all that time?" I can always count on Neo to hit me with a direct shot, no warning over the bow.

"I have tried to push harder and go faster to make this healing happen. It's not helping. The old way of using fierce 'push harder' is not working. I have used anger to motivate, to push me harder, so I can accomplish more, but no longer. The anger now adds stress, experienced raw and unfiltered. I can no longer afford to do things the old way if I'm looking for genuine wellness."

"Sounds like you want to get rid of anger. That's a tall order. Lots of good reasons for keeping anger in the back pocket and pulling it out when it's needed." Neo is justifying his point.

I take a deep breath, and with an unusual calmness, reply, "I don't think I can get rid of it. I think it's a part of who I am. But I do think I have misused and abused the energy behind the anger. I always used the injustice connected to suffering and the objectification of others to inflame me. I have used this fire to fuel my motivation, to continue the good fight."

Neo retorts quickly, "Yeah man. Help the good guys and kill the bad guys – anger is good for that."

I shake my head, "There is an attacking edge to anger, but it is not an absolute quality of anger. Rather, it is a self-imposed one. I willingly choose to attack with anger. It is not necessary for wellness and I experience this attacking edge as harmful to my search for healing. I need to remove this self-imposed attack quality and embrace a transformed anger."

With a slight turn of the head in a little gesture of acknowledgment, Neo says, "Peace on Earth and good will to all, I get it. But anger is also good for helping me get my point across, get their attention."

"Not always, Neo. Powerful ideas have enough of a spark in them to kindle awakening in the hearts of all who can listen. All that the fire of anger does is obscure the discovery of that spark. While healing I need that spark, I need what's behind that spark, and using anger to incite just gets in the way."

As I walk over to the kitchen to cut up zucchini (there's always too much zucchini in New England, even in winter), I can see Neo crinkling as he wrestles with his thoughts about anger. As if a light bulb went off over Neo, he blurts, "Sometimes, I just want to blow off some steam. Anger is a good way doing that."

I respond, "Whenever I'm in one of those venting moods I also have this internal dialog that is filled with negative statements about people, about life, about past events. It's inner dialog that points fingers at 'he said this,' 'she did that,' 'not fair that this happened to me,' and 'I want this to go away.' The venting is filled with a lot of energy, almost a rush can go with it. In the past, it may have helped. But now, the emotional intensity of this venting is no longer healthy for me. And it can hurt people around me."

I take a sip of holiday cider and then continue. "There is a different way to look at how to use the energy behind anger, the energy of perceived injustice. It is a way of taking that energy to focus it solely on solutions – not on people, not on personal injury, not on personal feelings. Every problem is a solution waiting to happen. Shifting the focus of the energy toward constructive change changes the nature and quality of anger."

Neo has been tapping lightly on the table for the last 30

seconds, and now he jumps in. "You will need that anger if your life is threatened – or the lives of your children or grandchildren. You'll need that anger energy then for sure."

Taking a deep breath after a lengthy pause, I say, "Most of us are not faced with actual life-threatening situations. There are places in the world where such threats are real, and in those situations, people need to act in a way that preserves both life and humanity. But for most of us, it is the perceived threat or illusions of threat that enters our lives. Remove the illusions and you remove the need for anger to function in this manner. Anger is reframed, transformed."

Neo nods, "So the gift of forgiveness, tolerance, and patience is in keeping with the holiday season. It's a good gift for yourself and for others."

Neo and I agree. Reframing is a powerful tool to help facilitate positive change. No more anger motivating me to push harder and faster. Let it go! It's OK if it took four months to go from zero to sixty.

The Relationship of PTSD and PD

I was out gathering flowers: peach tulips and blue orchids. It was a beautiful sun-kissed day, filled with thoughts about where I would discover new blooms in the garden. Out of nowhere, a chasm opened beneath my feet, plummeting me a long way down into unknown depths. Jagged rocks and outcrops tore at me and bruised every part of me. Now mind you, this was part of a virtual game experience, but it still took a toll.

Days with PD are like this. It's sunny. I stop to smell the roses, have positive expectations, and then something inflames my PD symptoms. Like falling into that virtual chasm, I am forced to stop doing what I planned and go in a totally different direction. I call it "PD forcing," and it is happening more often these days.

I had a doctor tell me, "All Vietnam vets have PTSD." It's an over-generalization that I don't agree with. However, a 2019 study has suggested that military veterans with post-traumatic stress disorder (PTSD) or who experienced a traumatic brain injury have more than double the risk of rapid eye movement (REM) sleep behavior disorder. REM has also been implicated as a risk factor for Parkinson's disease. Researchers at the VA Portland Health Care System and Oregon Health and Science University plan to explore the association of Parkinson's among veterans with REM sleep behavior disorder (RBD). "This is important because, in the general population, RBD has been linked to Parkinson's disease, and RBD often precedes classic symptoms of Parkinson's by years," Miranda Lim, M.D., Ph.D., a staff physician at the VA, and the study's senior author, said.[128]

A 2017 study has shown patients with PTSD had an elevated risk of developing PD in later life. They recommended further studies to clarify the exact relationship between PTSD and PD and investigate whether the prompt intervention for PTSD may reduce this risk.[129]

To some extent, I think that PTSD can be brought on (or exacerbated by) facing Parkinson's daily symptoms. The PD symptoms and expressions of PTSD and PD progression are also similar: irritability and angry outbursts (with little or no

---

[128] "Veterans with PTSD or Brain Injury at Risk of Sleep Disorder That Might Signal Parkinson's, Study Finds." By Alice Melao, "News," published on Parkinson's News Today, October 16, 2019.

[129] Yee-Lam E. Chan, Ya-Mei Bai, Ju-Wei Hsu, Kai-Lin Huang, Tung-Ping Su, Cheng-Ta Li, Wei-Chen Lin, Tai-Long Pan, Tzeng-Ji Chen, Shih-Jen Tsai, Mu-Hong Chen, "Post-traumatic Stress Disorder and Risk of Parkinson Disease: A Nationwide Longitudinal Study," The American Journal of Geriatric Psychiatry, Volume 25, Issue 8, 2017, Pages 917-923, ISSN 1064-7481, https://doi.org/10.1016/j.jagp.2017.03.012.

provocation), verbal or physical aggression toward people or objects when the frustrations of physical or mental challenges become "up close and personal," reckless or self-destructive behavior, hypervigilance, exaggerated startle response, problems with concentration and sleep disturbances.[130]

Living with ever-increasing and debilitating progression of PD symptoms can be traumatic. Coping with the symptoms, we seek a variety of escape modes, and old habits no longer work.[131] Trauma doesn't just come from being in military combat. It can come from being in combat with a chronic disease. PTSD is the result of a maladaptive coping response to traumatic memories. This is different than what happens initially with the exaggerated stimuli input. The exaggerated input is tied to the development of coping skills but they are not maladaptive. This means they are not interfering in the quality of life. In the case of this author, the opposite is true. Coping skills have led to an improvement of quality of life.

The PD thief that keeps coming back – unexpected, unwanted, and unforgettable – continues to steal away another skill or capability. I never know where the next chasm will open beneath my feet. I realize that as I worked on the physical healing this year, I could hear the suffering more clearly. After making progress with managing my anger, every day is the fear of being traumatized again. "What next?" I retreated into a cocoon, a lounge chair, and a sedentary life. Up until now, I didn't think the PTSD label fit. The PD thief, however, continues to be a source for traumatization and just

---

[130] Center for Substance Abuse Treatment (US). *Trauma-Informed Care in Behavioral Health Services*. Rockville (MD): Substance Abuse and Mental Health Services Administration (US); 2014. (Treatment Improvement Protocol (TIP) Series, No. 57.) Exhibit 1.3-4, DSM-5 Diagnostic Criteria for PTSD. Available from:
https://www.ncbi.nlm.nih.gov/books/NBK207191/box/part1_ch3.box16/
[131] "Going from Zero to 60 in 4 Months." Dr. C. "Possibilities with Parkinson's," Published on Parkinson's News Today, December 20, 2019.

as powerful as my military experiences in Vietnam.

The sedentary life is a dangerous one, but I needed time to heal. When I finally ventured out into the world, I didn't feel safe because of the PTSD of PD and the loss of vision. Interacting with the world provides a regular stream of, "You can't do this anymore." It is often overwhelming, and it is happening more often these days.

I know it's time to leave my cocoon of safety. I know the world is not always painted with the dark palette of the PD thief. The sun still sends her shimmering fairies to dance on the lake ripples. Trees still whisper melodies in harmony with the wind. Yes, it is hard to motivate myself to move and engage after being sedentary for many months. But my gardens will bloom again, and so will I. Like the chartreuse spring bulbs bursting through the soil, signs of wellness are showing up in my life: muscle injuries healed, appetite returning, months spent retraining my eyes to see differently,[132] a drop in pain, and a significant decrease in the length and duration of vertigo. The sedentary time was focused on healing, but now it is time for me to leave the chair.

Moving out of a sedentary life isn't easy, but the wellness map helps. There is nothing good about the sedentary life when prolonged. It is time now to get up and show up for the next destination on the map. I need to beat back the PD thief and his sidekick, PTSD. It is time for me to do that.

---

[132]"Living Well with Low Vision." Dan Roberts, reviewed by Jennifer Galbraith, O.D., published on Living Well with Low Vision, September 7, 2005

In Search of Acceptance: Mumbles, Fumbles, and Stumbles

Researchers have said that combining acceptance with meditation works better than meditation alone.[133] Sounds like a fantastic idea. I've been having trouble with meditation ever since the ruin of stagnation. Maybe if I search for and discover how to combine acceptance with meditation,[134] that it will make a difference in my pursuit of well-being. The research supports this.[135]

It's winter and we are barricaded in our house by six-foot snowbanks. Getting out to my sanctuary in the garden and forest is almost impossible. Without a physical sanctuary, it's difficult for my mind to find peace. But I'm going to give this "acceptance" idea serious consideration. Family members

---

[133] Lindsay, Emily K. and John David Creswell. "Mindfulness, acceptance, and emotion regulation: perspectives from Monitor and Acceptance Theory (MAT)." *Current Opinion in Psychology*, Volume 28, 2019, Pages 120-125, ISSN 2352-250X, https://doi.org/10.1016/j.copsyc.2018.12.004.

[134] Desbordes, G., Negi, L. T., Pace, T. W. W., Wallace, B. A., Raison, C. L., & Schwartz, E. L. (2012). "Effects of mindful-attention and compassion meditation training on amygdala response to emotional stimuli in an ordinary, non-meditative state." *Frontiers in Human Neuroscience, 6*, 292.

Alberts, H. J. E. M., Schneider, F., & Martijn, C. (2012). "Dealing efficiently with emotions: acceptance-based coping with negative emotions requires fewer resources than suppression." *Cognition & Emotion, 26*(5), 863–870.

[135] Hayes, S. C., Strosahl, K. D., & Wilson, K. G. (1999). *Acceptance and commitment therapy: an experiential approach to behavior change*. New York: The Guilford Press.

Instead of the whole book try this shorter version: https://pro.psychcentral.com/child-therapist/2019/09/brief-summary-of-the-6-core-processes-of-acceptance-and-commitment-therapy-act/

More supportive science: Wang, Yuzheng et al. "Effect of Acceptance versus Attention on Pain Tolerance: Dissecting Two Components of Mindfulness." *Mindfulness* vol. 10,7 (2019): 1352-1359.

have said, "You're disabled. Accept it and get on with your life." Can't be that hard. I just need to say to myself, "Accept your chronic disease, and accept your vision loss." With a pint of ice cream in hand, I repeat this acceptance mantra. Half an hour later, with the ice cream gone, I feel nothing from the mantra. But there is a touch of pleasure from the ice cream devoured.

It just doesn't seem right saying to myself that I accept everything about my chronic disease and vision loss. Repeating the "mantra" turned me into a zombie. It's just an outright lie. I don't accept everything as it currently stands because I believe that the pursuit of wellness contains vast undiscovered territory.

My wellness map is only the beginning of the journey. For me to accept everything about my condition feels like resignation, as if I'm giving up and allowing life with PD to just take over. There must be a better way for me to embrace acceptance.

Pacing the floor and fidgeting with my tablet and videogame, I try something different. "I accept that I am responsible for managing how the disease affects my behaviors and how those behaviors affect my quality of life." This is my new mantra. I repeat these words as often as possible between smashing monsters on my video games. After an hour of mantra repetition, I find no new levels of peace. But I did go up a couple of levels in my game, and that left me with a touch of happiness.

Acceptance has this utopic vision connected to its construct. If I can drink successfully from the cup of acceptance, the elixir will help heal my troubled being. But I don't even have my hands on the cup – half empty or half full! I put the videogame down, and now I'm just pacing the floor wringing my hands and mumbling. With a drink in one hand, I reach for a bowl of chips and miss – CRASH! – bowl and chips scatter on the floor.

Mrs. Dr. C. comes into the room with a worried look. "It's OK, I can clean that up for you." I respond, "No, I'll get it." I turn without thinking, relying on my body to remember how to move, reaching too quickly to grab a broom, but my body doesn't engage as fast as my mind and I stumble. Mrs. Dr. C. smiles and says calmly, "You seem a little out of sorts. What's going on?"

I look away from her and my head hangs low. "I've been struggling with this idea of acceptance. I just can't accept everything."

Giving me a light hug, Mrs. Dr. C. consoles me. "You do tend to overthink things. Just start small. Start with something easy, like accepting mumbles, fumbles, and stumbles. You can say, 'I accept these things will happen in my life. I will do what I can to decrease their impact. Ultimately, I must accept that these things are happening and will continue to happen.'"

I collapse in my chair almost dumbfounded. "You're right. Acceptance doesn't have to be this wave that washes everything clean. It's not about perfection. It's about small baby steps. It's a calm meditative acceptance of those small steps – mumbles, fumbles, and stumbles."

I sink back into my chair and repeat my new mantra between deep meditative breaths, "I accept mumbles, fumbles, and stumbles. I'm doing all that I can using my wellness map." There is a revelation that gentle peace is discovered in this special combination of acceptance mantra and meditative breath. The two seem to enhance each other, acting as catalysts to the other. It's an unusual sensation, a soothing comfort lasting for hours, that I had not discovered prior to the investigation for this essay. This is the path of possibilities that runs through my wellness map and leads me to moments of well-being – despite the chronic disease.

Watch out for the Good Days!

"Oh my gosh! The presentation was amazing. And I'm not just saying that because I'm your partner."

It was my first presentation about my experience with Parkinson's and it flowed smoothly. It had been a long time since I was in front of an audience, reaching out and connecting. Time was suspended, and I found my bliss again. I was bounding around the house like a young boy who got his first bike for Christmas. Riding the wave of unbridled enthusiasm, I said, "Now there is nothing stopping Dr. C from becoming successful!" I turned my head slightly and gave Mrs. Dr. C. a wry smile. And she gave me "the look" that suggests tempering the emotional "high" to avoid a crash later.

The next day, I crashed emotionally and physically because I let the excitement of the day run free without restraint to the point where the consequences were not healthy – the opposite of what the bliss experience should provide. I know I'm supposed to watch out for those good days because they will sneak up on me.

Threshold management is the practice of calming emotional input prior to thinking or reacting to that input. This calming practice helps prevent a buildup of emotional energy that can toss someone over the threshold. My previous essays have focused on emotions like irritability and anger. Getting overly excited about good things in life can create just as many problems. PD patients can experience this "emotional lability." If I keep threshold management practices in place during a good day, then the crash doesn't have negative impacts.

Exploring the possibility for discovering new early PD symptoms continues to be of major concern to me. It might be that in some PD patients emotional signal input is heightened, or the normal filtering mechanisms of the brain are diminished and thus the emotional signal appears heightened. PD patients can have one or more of the following: depression, anxiety, and/or impulse control.

With the recent increase in severity of my PD symptoms, I now get surges of depression, anxiety, and an annoying startle response. Absurdly, I got startled by a very loud crash from a blob of shampoo falling from soapy hair and hitting the shower floor. Prior to PD, I had no history of these exaggerated emotional responses. Exaggerated input on good days is my new life. I feel like I've gone past the borders of my wellness map. I am taking my explorer's machete out of the toolkit and blazing a path to new wellness practices.

In addition to practicing threshold management to keep excitement from running rampant, there are two other practices that help me stay balanced during the good times. The first is, "Don't chase after the blissful feelings." The second is, "Accept the good day as it presents and channel your energy accordingly." Part of what fuels excitement running rampant is chasing after it because I want it to last longer.

There is an interesting phenomenon that occurs during good days: my PD symptoms are less severe, sometimes strikingly so. I noticed this also with other pleasure-related experiences, like enjoyment from creativity, or an excellent movie, or a romantic evening with Mrs. Dr. C. The positive effects from bliss are more powerful and longer lasting. Even so, all my chasing results in negative consequences. Chasing things that feel good is composed of habitual thought and habitual action. It can be changed.

We all have different things that we do that help us to feel better. Maybe it's a hot shower with the warm water massaging sore muscles. It could be a good book at night where we can escape into the writer's world. It becomes a problem when chasing after feeling good replaces constructively changing thought and action to become more open to experiencing well-being moments. This is not easy.

It's not about perfect abstinence. It's about paying attention to that big neon sign that says, "Caution! Chasing risk ahead."

One of my observations regarding human change is that you can't change something into nothing. If you're seeking to remove a behavior, for example, chasing after "feel good," it is quite difficult to be successful if you're just asking the behavior to be gone. Once the behavior is gone, then there is a void, an empty space where a thought or action response used to go. If another thought or action is not put in that void, then the old thought and action will return quicker than you can snap your fingers. Fortunately, "seeking acceptance" offers us just what we need: the good days can be handled just in the same way we handle the bad ones. We calmly accept what the good days bring in the same way that we calmly accept the bad ones. It's a pathway full of possibilities.

Movement Fluidity Improves for Parkinson's Patients when in Formal Settings

"My husband wobbles a lot when getting up from the sofa. I'm afraid he will fall. What can we do about that?" asked the patient's wife at my last presentation to a PD support group. Turning to her husband, I asked if he would mind standing up. He did so quite gracefully. A slight hesitation accompanied motor initiation, but there was no severe wobbling. This provided an opportunity for me to explain to the audience how movement fluidity with Parkinson's disease can be improved under formal settings.

This is not new information to me, but it was to the audience. I had heard stories from Parkinson's patients that their motor symptoms would have less of a disabling effect when they were in a formal setting, like entertaining company or presenting in front of a group, versus informal settings like sitting at home on the sofa watching TV. Unfortunately, the doctor's office is often viewed as a formal setting by the patient, and when asked by the provider to stand or sit, I perform well, occasionally with a little hesitation but no serious wobbling. But at home, moving through space and time is a quite different display of uncoordinated arms and legs.

Motor hesitation accompanying motor initiation is common for PD patients under both formal and informal settings. This motor hesitation can be followed by wobbling, instability, and even stumbling when moving from sitting to walking, particularly in informal settings. Knowing this to be true is of great benefit because we can use that information to open more possibilities with Parkinson's disease, especially in the early stages.

Why does this happen? In previous essays, I have talked about autopilot and scenario looping. We don't have to think about walking. It's an overlearned motor sequence which is stored in memory, accessed by the autopilot, and tied into the scenario looping process. Those of us who have Parkinson's disease experience scenario looping breakdowns and a broken autopilot. This means that we cannot rely on our bodies to automatically (using autopilot), and smoothly, move from a sitting position to walking. The autopilot is broken, so there's a good chance you're going to see wobbling, instability, and stumbling – particularly in informal settings. This is because in informal settings, our minds tend to be focused on other things. We habitually assume that our body will automatically get up off the sofa and proceed to walk into the kitchen without us having to do anything special. But this is no longer the case in PD patients. What formal settings have shown us is that when we pay extra attention to our movements, they can become less problematic.

Falling is a serious concern, and we need to do anything and everything we can to decrease the possibility of this

155

happening in our lives. Mindful movements can be incorporated into our lives in more situations than just the formal.

It may seem strange, but I've begun to "perform" with my movements daily. It's sort of like doing Tai Chi or dancing each time I get up out of the chair, every time I walk from the bathroom to the living room, every time I get out of the bed.

The Big and Loud program[136] begins to touch upon mindful movement. When we incorporate mindful movement into our own lives, it needs to be personal, intentional, and eventually common practice. Mindful movements can be tailored to fit into our own lifestyle. It took me about six months of daily practice before mindful movement became a regular part of how I move around in the world. Mindful movement turns the informal into the formal.

Using mindful movements to turn the informal into the formal starts with a pause. Before I move from one position to another, like moving from sitting on the sofa to walking into the kitchen, I pause. Into that pause I put my practice of focusing my attention on every little movement of feet, arms, legs. In addition, the movement is slower, slightly exaggerated, and perceptually (at least in my mind) graceful – like Tai Chi or dancing. Remember, perfection is not the goal here; it's an improved quality of life. It takes some time for mindful movement to become a regular part of daily life, and thus have an impact on quality of life, but it is well worth the effort.

---

[136] Learn about LSVT BIG, who it helps, and how it differs from other physical/occupational therapies. https://www.lsvtglobal.com/LSVTBig

Moving Tips: Are You Crazy? Conversation with Neo

"What? You're moving again? Are you insane?" Neo exclaims.

"I've been called many things, yet still retain my sanity. I hope to do so through this stressful process of moving," I answer back.

"How do you plan on doing that? You're giving up your sanctuary!" Neo continues.

"The beauty of this physical sanctuary can be recreated, and we carry the rest with us," I reply. "Yes, there is a sense of loss that is made more difficult by the recent changes in my physical abilities. But the move is necessary for creating a higher quality of life for me, and for Mrs. Dr. C."

I put on my winter protective gear as I brave the snow and head for the ice-covered trees. Time to feed our menagerie of wild birds. The chickadees swoop and dart to the feeders so close to me I can hear the beating of their wings. The still remoteness allows the soft symphony of feathers in the wind to fill my ears and soothe my soul. "Dr. C." found his voice within the stillness. It was a time of introspection, of contemplation, of fear of the future, confronted by the courage to accept the progression of a chronic disease, and the addition of a debilitating loss of vision. After all that good healing work, is now the right time to move?

There will always be doubts. I loved this place. It will be hard to leave this serene sanctuary. Here, my mind came to understand the challenges so many people face with chronic disease. It was a time to learn to write and communicate the fears, hopes, challenges, and possibilities. Now is the time to be closer to an area that can help Dr. C. share the message with more people. It will be stressful.

Neo hesitates, pondering, "So, this move is about 'Dr. C.?'"

"Mostly," I reply. "It is also about moving where it is warmer, where garden time is longer. The garden sanctuary here is only available for a limited time. I need more sanctuary time to diminish the effects of this disease progression.

"Access to healing resources is also severely limited if we continue to live here," I say quite firmly. With a partner who also has a chronic disease, the effort to maintain good health takes a toll on both of us. We spend as many days in 'recovery' as we do scheduling medical appointments, rescheduling due to bad weather conditions, driving for hours to attend appointments, and then returning home, usually completely exhausted. We lose several days of what could be dedicated to productive projects just surviving through these ordeals. We need to be closer to medical services.

We have also found that support from the community is important. 'Dr. C.' cannot simply think about what rambles around in his own head. He needs to be out in the community to help others, and to find encouragement and caring. It is relationships with others that brings about Dr. C.'s voice in his writing. The move will help Dr. C.'s healing circle expand."

Neo scoffs at that notion. "Given the number of moves you and Mrs. Dr. C. have undertaken, you would think you would be experts by now! What, you think there are obstacles you haven't faced before?"

"Yes, Neo, and you should know them as well. No longer are we able to consider a house without access and safety features. We are learning that we must allow ourselves double or triple the amount of time to do anything strenuous. And, it seems, a lot of any kind of physical movement is strenuous. Moving stressors take a serious toll now because stress is experienced more intensely due to heightened emotional input."[137]

It's not easy to justify needing additional time to rest. Both of us are guilty of trying to push through it. That was the old way, and it doesn't work anymore. Emotional thresholds are easily reached during the stress of moving, thresholds that overwhelm both of us. The move heightens everything that Parkinson's patients face even on a good day. The best tip we can offer is to take breaks often and <u>early</u> in the threshold management process. Meditate <u>as soon</u> as moving stressors begin to show their ill effects. Repeat as many times as needed during the day.

Finding reference material addressing the needs of Parkinson's disease patients when they are moving to a new home is difficult. We put together a list of links to help Parkinson's patients who are moving.[138] Neo and I will chat again, sharing more tips, as we head to our new urban home location close to our granddaughters.

Big Boys Don't Whine

"Oh, poor me. I have lost so much." I moan, hanging my head down and shuffling my feet.

Mrs. Dr. C. glances up from her book. "Did you say something, dear?"

"Just another rough period," I say with an affect as flat as the tarmac at LaGuardia Airport. It's a personal choice to continue working on acceptance without the self-pity. Some days are better than others, but I resist the cacophony of emotions: grief, sadness, anger, frustration, and anxiety.

---

[137] Blonder, Lee X, and John T Slevin. "Emotional dysfunction in Parkinson's disease." *Behavioural neurology* vol. 24,3 (2011): 201-17. doi:10.3233/BEN-2011-0329

[138] See list at https://www.drc.life/tip%20for%20moving.html

Mostly, I don't believe their narrative.

I don't want to whine about an inner dialog that is based on old voices from a dysfunctional family past. I replace the "whine" with "I'm defining." Not, "I'm OK, you're OK," or "Go to your happy place and you will be all better," or the Pollyanna philosophy of, "Really, I'm doing fine with it all. I really am... believe me." Instead, it's an honest assessment that the glass is half full and half empty at the same time. If I am whining, then I am not defining all the possibilities to be found.

Moving to a new house and new location causes stress. So far, my threshold management practices help about 90% of the time. There is no room for whining in my schedule these days. I don't have enough personal resources to manage my chronic disease and finish all the tasks needed to prepare for our move. Realizing this did cause some internal dissonance, my bemoaning the situation, but mostly because I didn't know how to ask for help. So, I felt trapped – and that can get dark very quickly.

I mentioned that I am at the edge of my wellness map, an explorer surveying the wild frontiers of an unexplored wisdom regarding living well with a chronic disease. I ran out of answers. Again stuck.

Wait! Maybe other people have written about living with a chronic disease? Why have I been so slow to grasp the obvious? Or, as Mrs. Dr. C. says, "Uh duh..." To my surprise, I found many books. I dove into one called *Dancing with Elephants* by Jarem Sawatsky.[139]

As the author says, the book is not about frolicking with pachyderms. It is about how we, as individuals and as a community, address the elephant in the room – the chronic

---

[139] Sawatsky, Jarem. *Dancing with Elephants: Mindfulness Training for Those Living With Dementia, Chronic Illness or an Aging Brain* (How to Die Smiling Book). Red Canoe Press, 2017.

disease. The author says that most of us don't know how to offer help or how to ask for it.

I learned something through all of this. Asking someone for help is most likely to be successful when the request is fully understood, joyfully accepted, and matches the abilities of the person giving the help. Sounds like common sense. But the answers are not straightforward.

Success is tied to the degree of fit between the one in need, the tasks to be done, and the talents of the other. This degree of fit has several parameters shaping its outcome. I have spent more than three decades examining this idea. Yet, when it came to the simple task of asking for help, I was stymied. Maybe it is like when guys don't ask for directions, drive around for hours "mansplaining" they are not lost, with a partner fuming in the passenger seat. The problem is the cost of being lost inside my chronic disease has too high a price. I had to ask for help.

The result: my brother's help was instrumental in getting us ready to move, my stress level decreased – reflecting to Mrs. Dr. C. an improved ability to deal with the stress of moving. It is the first time in my life where I could not, due to the chronic disease, complete tasks by myself that were important to the well-being of me and Mrs. Dr. C. The turmoil that swirls around even considering asking for help is linked to self-image.

One of the problems of chronic disease is that it tears at the flesh of self-image. In the beautifully written book *When Breath Becomes Air*,[140] the author speaks about the shifting sands of identity when the tsunami of chronic disease keeps knocking you down. With a Ph.D. in rehabilitation counseling, I know about adaptability, about making accommodations that are adjustments to the physical and cognitive changes of

---

[140] Kalanithi, Paul. *When Breath Becomes Air*. First edition. New York: Random House, 2016.

chronic disease. I just wasn't ready to dive under the tsunami, into the deep water of the human psyche, to find ways of bolstering a new identity. I'm not a particularly good swimmer.

So, I'm replacing whining with defining those things most important to a self-identity that has meaning and purpose. This includes asking for help. Mrs. Dr. C. is smiling at me.

Brain Therapy for Parkinson's

For my Ph.D. research, I wanted to examine in more detail the processes by which humans move from traumatic injury, like TBI, to a place of well-being. My clinical experience led me to consider two things that people drew upon. First, they drew upon cognitive processes when recovering from trauma. Second, the recovery process was helped by the relationship between the injured and those who are deemed healing practitioners. I witnessed a special kind of relationship that directly affects healing. It is this healing relationship that became the focal point for my Ph.D.

But I never let go of my deep belief in neural plasticity and our ability to cultivate our own neural sprouting. Little did I know then that I'd be applying healthy doses of brain therapy fertilizer to my own neural branches in fighting the progression of Parkinson's disease.

PD is complex in presentation and it's difficult to find a set of symptoms, along with their progression, that fit anything more than about half of the population of PD patients. It's been frustrating trying to advance my own cerebral rehab in the face of unclear guideline. Whatever I choose as brain activities each day is going to affect my health. To decide which brain activities are best, I need some clear brain therapy guidelines.

Throughout my essays, I've been talking about creating a wellness map. This is a metaphor for brain therapy. Much of what I have written is tied to a brain model based on functional neuroanatomy of the connections between the prefrontal cortex and the thalamus (see the link reference lists at www.drc.life). This is graphically illustrated in "Brain Therapy Theory for Parkinson's Disease." The figure shows a "Grand Central Station" where sensory stimulus input comes in and gets routed back out to the appropriate destination. There are several "most popular" destinations: motor sequencing autopilot, making and carrying out plans, memory – short-term and long-term – and actions/thoughts that are deemed needing more immediate attention (often emotion laden).

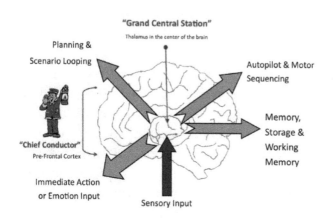

Brain Therapy Theory for Parkinson's Disease

GraphicDesign by Corey Inlsington

Overseeing all of this is the "conductor." The conductor's main responsibility is to make sure that the most important things get on the tracks out of the "Grand Central Station" before less important things. The theory proposed here is that scenario looping breakdowns, a malfunctioning autopilot, and exaggerated stimuli input are happening with information coming out of the "Grand Central Station." It is information that got on the tracks without conductor intervention.

This theory proposes that these "conductor to Grand Central Station malfunctions" are major contributors to PD symptoms. If we can decrease the effects of scenario looping breakdowns, the malfunctioning autopilot, and exaggerated emotional stimuli, then the effects of Parkinson's disease should be less.

There is a second part to this theory which states that the conductor is still able to direct traffic out of "Grand Central Station." Add to this that neural plasticity is a process still available in our senior years of life, albeit slower. The conductor resides in the front part of our brain (frontal lobe), and is often referred to as "executive functioning." I think this term is too broad in its definition and lacks the specificity needed for me to design brain therapy. The success of my personal brain rehabilitation depends on my success in training the conductor. This is one of those frontiers of wisdom exploration.

I have been hesitant about putting such an immature theory into the public domain, but I was encouraged by short few paragraphs in the book by neurosurgeon Paul Kalanithi in his book, *When Breath Becomes Air*.[141] He describes performing deep brain stimulation (DBS) on a Parkinson's patient. In the middle of the procedure, the doctor needed to shift the electrode a few millimeters within the thalamus. The patient was complaining of intense mood surges that had no

---

[141] Ibid.

connection to context, but a small shift of the electric stimulus provided relief. What intrigued me was that the stimulation of the thalamus triggered surges of exaggerated mood that had no link to content. I've termed them SEM (surges of exaggerated mood) attacks. It was exciting to discover that a tiny shift and the electrode was all that was needed, and poof, emotion stable tremor reduced. I thought, "Perhaps I can train my brain to do its own natural version of DBS?"

Stress, Emotion, and Brain Therapy: Conversation with Neo

"Hey Doc, you don't look so good. Like a walking zombie." Neo says with genuine concern in his voice.

I let out a bigger sigh than usual. "This move to halfway across the continent is unusually difficult. The Surges of Exaggerated Mood (SEM) attacks are worse with the stress. While preparing to move, I am practicing mindful movement as often as possible and supporting Mrs. Dr. C. through the process; I am also practicing brain therapy to moderate these SEM attacks. I feel like 'the walking dead' because I'm still not fully recovered from the 'ruin of stagnation.'"

Neo snorts. "You have always been your worst enemy, pushing yourself to exhaustion. Maybe the old ways aren't working for you anymore. You need to take a good dose of your own advice!"

Neo always surprises me by how he cuts to the heart of the matter. "Absolutely!" I respond. "I have to find a new way. That's what this brain therapy is about. It's a new way of monitoring and changing how I live with the symptoms of chronic illness, especially the SEM attacks."

"Never heard of such a thing. How can you prove this 'brain therapy' works for anybody but yourself?" Neo doesn't completely discount my idea, but he's not buying it 100%.

"I am in the hypothesis clarification stage right now. Not ready yet to explore the therapeutic efficacy of brain therapy. We are still exploring the idea that the brain has a built in 'conductor' which can be trained to moderate the SEM attacks." I respond with confidence.

Neo ponders this idea. "Have you found any clues that might indicate what this might look like?"

My thoughts start flowing. "It's preliminary, but perhaps brain therapy will include wellness mapmaking using CHRONDI, threshold management, mindful movement, a psychological awareness called high self-monitoring,[142] and regular involvement in new and novel problem-solving."

Neo's concentration is glazing over. "That's a lot for a person to try to do when they have to battle a chronic disease, support Mrs. Dr. C. with a chronic disease, and deal with the stress of moving."

"Getting overwhelmed happens to me every day. If I can practice high self-monitoring, it helps to keep things in check. It's not about perfection, but rather calm reflection. No matter what's in front of me, I try to calmly reflect on my perceptions prior to acting. On the good days I don't revert to the 'old ways' of thinking. But on the bad days the old ways still get me in trouble."

Neo responds with a sense of authority. "And what is Mrs. Dr. C. doing through all your efforts?"

"I wouldn't be able to do a lot of what I do without her. She has her own medical issues – her 'demons,' she calls them. She has had to make a lot of adjustments to her life at the same time I've been adjusting to mine. Most of the time, she says she can monitor my actions and knows when I'm not doing

---

[142] Gangestad, S. W., & Snyder, M. (2000). "Self-monitoring: Appraisal and reappraisal." *Psychological Bulletin, 126*(4), 530–555. https://doi.org/10.1037/0033-2909.126.4.530

well. It's the times when the SEM attacks occur seemingly out of nowhere and with no provocation. That's the hard part, but one of our strengths as a couple is we've always been able to talk through most anything. We work together on not harboring hurt feelings when the medical issues create problems – unexpected or expected. We talk, we adjust, we share, and we keep walking together through all of what we are both experiencing."

I pause, taking a bite of scrumptious peppermint chocolate pie provided by friends. "It's easy to get overwhelmed, but I remind myself it's just chemistry while I put the brain therapy to work. I am having to do this multiple times a day. The good news – the brain therapy program is helping. I deeply believe the brain is designed to do this and I can strengthen its natural ability as conductor. I'm still in the early stages of discerning the details, and a long way from teaching others how to do it."

Neo nods. "I think you're onto something here. I look forward to hearing more. Hopefully, your readers will provide informative comments and compassionate support for your continued journey into the frontiers of chronic disease rehabilitation. Oh, and by the way, you might just give Mrs. Dr. C. an extra hug today."

Going Numb, Going Nowhere

Sobbing, tears streaming, she throws her arms around me, "I just can't take one more thing (sobs, sniffs). I am totally overwhelmed. All the things I need to attend to are flying around me, and as I try to grasp onto one, I come away empty." She rests within my embrace and slowly the storm subsides. Lying next to her is like being in the middle of a tornado. Toto and the Wicked Witch share the violent winds of her emotional upheaval as I watch her life swirl around her.

I too feel overwhelmed and have little room for any additional feeling from any source. I want to jump in the car and drive away to some greener pasture, but I find that there is no place away from myself except that which I can create. Then, as if someone dropped a house on me, I shift into the altered state of being numb.

During my years of clinical practice, I saw many patients use the numb space as a form of protection during their recovery from a traumatic injury. They walk around glassy-eyed, seemingly lost in their own inner space. Conversations with them cover only the superficial generalities of daily life. I've always appreciated the need for people to create their own healing space, and I've never pushed against that space without informed consent. Right now, it seems that I need the numb space as part of staying healthy through the stress of moving.

The problem is that the numb space doesn't fit very well on me. Yes, in some ways the numb space is quiet and comforting. But it takes a lot of energy to put up all the blockades necessary to force that numb space into existence. The numb space should not be confused with the quiet stillness one can discover through diligent practice of meditation. Forcibly blocking out all feelings is not a quiet experience, and for me, it is difficult to maintain. Emotions have, and continue to be, an important way that I see the world, a third eye. Being legally blind, I need all the extra eyes I can get.

The numb space is also difficult on Mrs. Dr. C. She experiences it as a retreat from the intimacy and sharing that we have had for almost 50 years. With PD, I can't always join her on the simple errands of shopping, post office, or other chores that need to be attended. So, in addition to the loneliness of not doing things we used to do together, going numb widens that intimacy gap. Add to that all the swirling activity of selling and buying a home, preparing for the move and all the paperwork involved in relocating, and she feels even more distant.

When someone has a chronic illness, partners must work at and rely upon the underpinnings of their friendship, love, and communication. Like the tornado, the numb space threatens to tear all that apart. We both recognize it and make every effort to reach out and reconnect. She has often said that she doesn't want to be identified as a caretaker. In her eyes, being a "caretaker" requires a certain amount of distancing. Caretakers, she says, must separate from the "patient" in order to provide objective assessments. It is perhaps easier in some regards to not have a personal and intimate reaction to the emotional outbursts of SEM symptoms. It is difficult to not personalize the irritability, depression, or anxiety that PD patients exhibit. But as a partner, one has the history of knowing how the PD has changed emotions, but not the person underneath. The separation from the relationship into a "caretaker" role is much more rendering. There is a long history of good times and memories that can sustain the relationship. She feels that there is too high a risk in this separation that can be felt by the person wrestling with PD as a rejection of their self. It can very easily be construed as another "loss" when so many losses already exist. Being a partner means so much more, and Mrs. Dr. C. will not trade being a partner for a "caretaker." So, we work together, as we have done for decades, to give each other support through the storm.

I see the numb space as very temporary, an oasis, a break from the storm. It is not a destination because it leads nowhere. People get in trouble when they try to make the numb space a permanent destination visited daily, by whatever means. It may be harder to stay in touch with feelings during stressful times in life, but brain therapy is about taking the road less traveled and exercising your brain to build new neural connections. "Use it or lose it," remembering that going numb is going nowhere. It's an old way of coping that no longer works.

I think successful brain therapy will not only be built upon a sound theoretical foundation but will also include its delivery within supportive, healing, and growth-fostering relationships. Being in the numb space sabotages the healing relationship and all that it can contribute to successful brain therapy. The alternative to the numb space is shared space of friendship, support, love, and healing. It is a sacred space that defines the better part of humanity.

Expect the Unexpected

Travel beyond our homes is eerie right now with the onslaught of the coronavirus pandemic. We feel as if we're living a dystopian sci-fi film, with people in masks and gloves waving apocalyptic and often contradictory messages from so many sources.

My immune system isn't like it was when I was younger. I wear gloves for every outing. I wash my hands and apply antibacterial solutions. I wear a mask. But you just can't prepare for every possibility when traveling halfway across the continent. Expect the unexpected and the stress is more manageable.

Sitting for more than two hours is difficult for me. My muscles become rigid and painful. I resemble the Tin Man in *The Wizard of Oz*. Changing positions and making slight movements can ease the discomfort.

On the trip to go house hunting, we went by airplane. We had to accomplish a great deal in a short time, so driving was not an option. I had lots of room on the first flight due to a shortage of passengers. However, after switching planes for the second leg of the trip, I was in the middle seat. Despite the availability of other seating accommodations, an exceptionally large person decided to sit next to me in the aisle seat. Suddenly, I was restricted to my seat, unable to move or reposition my body as the muscle spasms started increasing. I couldn't really say, "Excuse me, but your sitting in that seat makes my body scream." How to explain what was going on, politely?

I ended up draping myself over Mrs. Dr. C. I focused on a lot of calming breath work. It's not like I can spend weeks in an airplane cabin simulator learning how to be at peace with a body that makes a lot of noise. Expect the unexpected.

I'm approved by my providers for medical marijuana use at home. I find it useful for pain management, as it helps to reduce rigidity and addresses pain receptors. When deciding to relocate, we chose our new home in an area that has legalized marijuana for both medical and recreational purposes. Recreational access was important because it will take time to get approved for medical marijuana after I establish residency. Federal law says I can't transport this medication across state borders – even for medical purposes. So, we had to find a dispensary during our house-hunting trip.

Because we had made our plans and reservations two months in advance, we anticipated the weather would be warmer there, as it usually is this time of year. We thought the dispensary "experience" would allow access quickly and efficiently, much as we have back home.

Instead, it was a four-hour wait in 40-degree weather with a brisk wind and only two fleece jackets for outerwear. That was Mrs. Dr. C. handling the unexpected – waiting in line, surrounded by a hundred other folks.

Back in the car, I was battling pain surges – sternocleidomastoid attacks (otherwise known as jaw-clenching) – every five to ten minutes over those four hours. Then, in the middle of that, I really, really had to find a restroom. I didn't know where I was, had never been there

171

before, and felt like every cell in my body was going to burst.

Looking out the car window across the parking lot, I saw a big sign: "Convention Center." Should be a restroom there, I surmised. I found one women's restroom, then two more women's restrooms down the hall. I said to myself, "What? Where's the men's restroom?"

I'm all for what architects identify as "potty parity" in their design elements. Potty parity is calculating the number of available restrooms by anticipating how many women and men will access public facilities. I know the number of women in most public accommodations greatly outnumber the men. But there is a time when a man needs to do what a man needs to do!

Parkinson's patients should *not* postpone their use of the restroom because of the additional discomfort that can happen when one tries to "hold it back for too long." I was quickly approaching that critical impasse as I found three women's restrooms and no men's restrooms. Doubled over and dashing at the same time (quite a sight), I saw a male custodian and thought, "Please, let him know where the men's room is." He did.

There is no way to prepare for this sequence of events. The unexpected will happen. The best we can do is embrace the unexpected, as well as the challenges and the opportunities that come with adapting to new situations.

Studies have shown that people who experience anticipated stressors have fewer physiological reactions[143] to those stressors than people who experience unanticipated stressors. For example, receiving electric shocks but not knowing when the shocks will be delivered will increase the stress reactions. The unexpected can ignite our fight-or-flight

[143] Meyer, Allison E., and John F. Curry. "Pathways from anxiety to stressful events: An expansion of the stress generation hypothesis." *Clinical Psychology Review*, Vol. 57, November 2017, Pages 93-116.

chemical maelstrom,[144] pushing us close to the threshold.

The unexpected carries with it the unknown, a "cloud of unknowing," a dissonance that drives demons into our desperation. Embracing the unexpected without a fear-based focus can decrease the effects of stress and shift the balance toward well-being and a positive outcome.

A positive outcome from our cross-country efforts: We found a home that would suit most of our needs. It was stressful but made easier by practicing brain therapy, including embracing the unexpected.

Shut In, Not Shut Out

Exhausted from the five-day trip to find a new home, my chronic disease forced me to be housebound for most of the week after my return. CHRONDI forcing, when the symptoms of a chronic disease force me to curtail life engagement outside the home, results in me becoming "locked down" inside my home. People throughout the nation are now being mandated into lockdown confinement to their homes due to the COVID-19 threat. This is probably a new and uncomfortable experience for many, but for those of us with a chronic disease, we have learned how to live in a locked down situation while not locking out the world. As a community, we have a pool of wisdom that can help people with this difficult adjustment.

Here is a list of tips I am using to help with this forced, but temporary, home confinement:

1) As needed, reach out to all available sources to secure food and shelter for you and your family.

---

[144] Neubauer, Andreas B., Joshua M. Smyth, Martin J. Sliwinski . "When you see it coming: Stressor anticipation modulates stress effects on negative affect." *Emotion*, April 2018, 18(3):342-354

2) Embrace with total commitment your responsibility to help curb the pandemic. Practice responsible social distancing along with hand and hard surface disinfecting. Respect the government's issuance of lockdown access if your area is affected.

3) Find ways to stay connected with co-workers, friends, and family while practicing social distancing. Use the Internet or texting, but don't stay glued to the screen. Pick one block of time each day to get updates from the news. Constant and relentless news will only serve to escalate emotions. Being informed is important. Being overwhelmed is not.

4) If you are working at home, realize that working at home is so much different than leaving the house and going to another building to work. Be patient with yourself and those around you while making the adjustments. Keep a regular schedule as much as you can. Being at home, it is often too tempting to work all the time. Make the time as you would for meals, family time, and activities. It takes time to adjust to the disruption of our "normal" work routine.

5) If you have other people living with you, more time must be spent on communications. Personal space becomes a priority. Set aside some place in the home that is your private space. Communicate that to the other people living with you.

6) Make time for threshold management. Emotions connected to the threat of serious infection can easily escalate to mass hysteria. It is quite easy to become emotionally overwhelmed, but when living in a lockdown environment, only you can quiet your own mind. Remember, this is temporary. Just put one foot in front of the other and stay safe.

7) This is an opportunity to engage in some activity at home that you always wanted to do but never had the

time to do it. I used my shut-in time to retrain my vision to automatically use e-centric viewing. This took hundreds of hours and helped me manage the shut-in time. Pick something that's important, something that you will stay engaged with during this virus crisis, something that will lift your spirits, and something that will improve your quality of life. You are locked down, but you are not locked out.

8) Maintain healthy life habits and try not to let the stress trigger a regression to old unhealthy habits – eat well, exercise, rest, and use the windows (patios, decks) to get a daily dose of sunshine and fresh air.

These are difficult times for each of us, for our communities, and for our country. Most people don't have the experience of being forced by a disease into home confinement. We, the community of people with chronic diseases, have a wealth of experience with such matters.

Social Distancing, Seeking Help, and Serenity

Sellers tore up the contract for our bid on a new home when they wanted to accept "better offer." We were now homeless. Well, almost. We have a committed sale of the home we are in and we had started thinking of the new place as "home," but that home was gone.

Some unexpected things hit hard no matter how well prepared we might be for the COVID-19 pandemic. The threat of being homeless is more than shocking. It can be a devastating blow to the psyche.[145] This threat is made even

---

[145] Goodman L., Saxe L., Harvey M. "Homelessness as psychological trauma. Broadening perspectives." *Am Psychol.* 1991 Nov;46(11):1219-25. doi: 10.1037//0003-066x.46.11.1219. PMID: 1772159.

more ominous to many people with the compounding dangers of contracting a terminal illness or being without financial means. These are scary times for everyone. But it is our job, each one of us, to maintain sanity in the middle of this pandemic chaos. In addition to Social distancing, Sanitizing, and Seeking help, let's add Serenity – the 4S pandemic safety program.

When we found out we could not buy that house, it was like being slapped in the face: Abrupt shock, nauseating, confusing, and an absence of connectedness. Home is sanctuary carved out to fit identity and purpose. Home cradles a lifetime of memories. Being without a home is to live in a state of groundlessness – a void lacking in both tangible and emotional connections. This groundlessness creates an absence of concrete information. It is a difficult state of consciousness, one which our minds seek relief from in any way possible.

The problem with the groundless state of consciousness is that, by its very nature, it is difficult to elucidate. It is not the numb state and is not the quiet mind. It is a state of consciousness where one sits with the discomfort of not knowing[146] and tries to calmly wait. If you frantically grasp for information within groundlessness, then the consciousness state shifts. In its place a flood of ill-informed emotions cascades. It is easy to attribute the uncomfortability of groundlessness to "he said," "she did," "they're not doing enough." We quickly blame the discomfort on something or someone external. We frenetically run around doing things we hope will make this hypothetical external cause go away.

---

[146] "The Cloud of Unknowing with the Book of Privy Counsel." Translated by Carmen Acevedo Butcher. Shambhala Publications. April 14, 2009.[147] American Psychological Association. "Stress Weakens the Immune System Friends, relaxation strengthens health." Published February 23, 2006.

Because we are blaming, and not serenely sitting, our thoughts, feelings and actions can make the situation worse – personally and for those around us.

One of the things that happens in response to the state of groundlessness is that people seek proof of future security. They want to be "sure" that nothing bad is going to happen to them in the future. This assuredness places the hope that the uncomfortability of groundlessness will dissipate. The sellers of the home we liked wanted proof, a guarantee, that we would buy their home regardless of our financial dependency on our current home's buyers. In a separate event, our son was seeking to sell his home. The buyers came back with an offer that included a termination clause if the pandemic worsened. These are illustrations of people trying to find a firmer footing within a terrain that is mostly groundless.

Immediately, or over time, we have each realized that having a chronic disease like Parkinson's means that we are never going to have absolute proof of future security. In both cases – of pandemic infection and chronic illness – we come to the realization that life is forever changed. We can choose to live a life of possibility, not only for personal well-being, but also for the well-being of others. In the face of groundlessness, we need to continue to make accommodations to a "new normal," communicate, and share compassion with our fellow humans.

We are all in this together and we can help each other by learning to sit serenely within a state of groundlessness as opposed to overreacting with a desperation to make the uncomfortability go away. Realistically, there is no proof that our future security will be guaranteed against the pandemic chaos or any other life situation. Chasing after such elusive proof often means we disregard people and actions that might help promote our well-being. Grasping after proof of future security just adds to stress, lowering our resistance to disease,[147] and adds to the stress of others around us.

Whether it is a pandemic or a chronic disease, we can keep ourselves in the moment to keep ourselves centered and safe.

Chocolate Chip Cookies vs. Toilet Paper: A Conundrum

If I were a hoarder, I would choose chocolate chip cookies over toilet paper. In a head-to-head match, chocolate chip cookies have many more benefits for coping with the pandemic crisis.

That soothing smell of a freshly baked cookie can't be matched by toilet paper, even the scented kind. A tray of warm, melt-in-your-mouth treats brings back memories of when the world was a simpler and safer place, and family and friends could share in the delight.

Imagine serving up a tray of warm toilet paper rolls. It just doesn't have the same good feeling. A well-made chocolate chip cookie is almost a survival staple. It covers several of my favorite food groups, including grains, nuts, and dairy. Toilet paper, although edible, doesn't fall under any food group. It is not recommended for oral intake.

Consuming chocolate chip cookies has the added benefit of psychological and emotional relief by lifting one's mood. There is relief in connection with acts preceding toilet paper use, but there is no causal link connecting toilet paper use and a long-lasting positive mood change. One quickly dismisses the experience and moves on with other more pressing issues.

When the Oracle in the movie *Matrix* tells the hero, who was extremely stressed, to sit and have a chocolate chip cookie to alleviate some of his anxiety, she was passing on the healing

---

[147] American Psychological Association. "Stress Weakens the Immune System Friends, relaxation strengthens health." Published February 23, 2006.

history that is baked into every homemade cookie. Toilet paper has nothing to match up with that.

The chocolate chip cookie is also famous. An ice cream flavor is named after it, a blue monster craves it, and Andie MacDowell thinks John Travolta smells like it in the movie *Michael.* The stardom of the cherished chocolate chip cookie blows toilet paper away. In lieu of other options, I'd hoard some extra chocolate chip cookies rather than extra toilet paper.

In my previous essay, I describe the "4S safety program," in which the final "S" stands for serenity. One of the steps that can be taken to help generate and pass on feelings of serenity is to maintain a lightness of being. One of the easiest ways to experience lightness of being is with humor.

Laughter is great medicine for people with Parkinson's and other chronic diseases, or for those just trying to survive each day of the COVID-19 outbreak. During these times, when the tender embraces of family and friends are absent, familiar stores and restaurants are closed, the comfort of routine is demolished, and doom and gloom run rampant through news broadcasts and almost all our conversations, it is essential to find moments of serenity.

Even now, in the middle of this pandemic, finding personal serenity is still possible – and bake up a batch of those cookies!

(Author's note: Nine months into the pandemic, cookie manufacturers report a 31% global increase in cookie consumption.[148])

---

[148] "Cookies a goodie of choice during pandemic, according to consumption report." Kevin Connor in the *Toronto Sun* online news. December 15, 2020.

Swarm of Waahdeefs: Conversation with Neo

Steam from my hot chocolate fogs my glasses. I almost miss Neo's opening comment: "How goes the move?"

I wipe my glasses. "We had to speed up the whole thing because of the pandemic. Trying to prepare for every possible concern during these unstable times has turned my brain to mush." Putting my glasses on, I feel Neo intensely listening. "I got overloaded and then..."

Neo interrupts, "Those are the classic symptoms of being swarmed by waahdeefs."

"Waah-what?" I ask.

Neo continues, "Oh yeah, they can be real nasty. They sneak into your mind and swirl around, wielding stingers of confusion and..."

My turn to interrupt. I shout, "Neo!"

"Oh yeah, sorry," Neo stammers. "A waahdeef is that 'what if' worry statement. When there is a swarm, it gets really messy – like a cerebral meltdown." Neo grins and says with confidence, "You know, what we need is a large can of waahdeef bug spray."

Laughing, I say, "I think I've got just the thing. Waahdeefs hate certainty. I don't have worry statements like, 'What if the sun doesn't come up tomorrow?' because, with a fair degree of certainty, I am sure the sun will come up tomorrow. Waahdeef swarm behavior is stimulated not by things that are certain, but rather things that are uncertain, like what is going to happen to us in a crisis."

Parkinson's patients have the waahdeef swarm effects also. Especially when they get that first diagnosis. The swarm returns with new symptoms or progression: What if I can't do something I used to be able to do? What if I need more help from family or friends? What is the next thing that is going to happen to me?

Neo clears his throat. "So, what you're saying is that if we can believe in the certainty of a future outcome, then it no longer becomes the target of a waahdeef swarm? Like using a can of bug spray?" Neo laughs.

"That's exactly right, Neo, and that bug spray is important when the waahdeefs are upon us." I sound like a general leading troops to battle.

Neo jumps to attention. "OK, general. Tell me how I can get my own can of bug spray."

So here are my suggestions:

- focus on what you *can* do (don't think about and don't talk about those things you cannot change)
- show up prepared for what you can do; remain motivated and engaged
- practice wellness behaviors including exercise, threshold management, and meditation
- keep the fear in check, knowing that the world has, and will continue to, survive crisis

Neo jumps in. "So, the bug spray instructions are to mix all that up and spray in the room? Then, hope for the best?"

"Yeah, that's about it," I answer, frankly.

Later that day, Neo returns and says, "I tried it and it helped a little. But there's this one pesky, buzzing idea and it's this: What if that one virus microbe that has survived the disinfectant onslaught manages to land on me? What can I do to stop it? There must be something I can do."

"That's a nasty one, Neo. That's the groundless variety of waahdeef. It's really difficult because nothing is more uncertain than groundlessness."

Neo, now showing a higher degree of frustration: "Are you telling me there isn't anything I can do to get rid of all these nasty waahdeefs?"

"All is not lost, Neo," I say with assured excitement. "This variety of waahdeefs has a short lifespan. We just need to sit and wait calmly until the cycle is over. And follow the best ideas to stay safe."

Neo collapses on the sofa. "Do all I can to keep myself and family safe. Keep the wellness program going. Be patient, relax, and wait until the waahdeefs are dead. Thanks... that helps."

Hungry for Hugs

I miss my support groups, the warm handshakes, and the genuine greeting, "How have you been?" Most of all, I miss hugs from my grandchildren. There is no technology that can replace their healing hugs.

We are social beings, and to thrive rather than just survive, we need healing contact with fellow human beings. As we consider phasing back into normal societal interactions, we should also phase in healing embraces in a manner that is safe for society.

Extended social isolation is not only detrimental to our economy, it also can have a negative impact on psychological and physical well-being. Premature babies who are provided with human touch thrive better than those who are not touched. Prisoner of war survivors provided with human contact from a friend during internment fared better than those without such contact. So much of human conversation is nonverbal and experienced face-to-face. The sharing of suffering and movement toward well-being is enhanced through physical contact, even a simple handshake.

For people with Parkinson's, tactile expression is often the most important means of communication. Some people have the "Parkinson's facial mask," which limits emotive expressions. Many people wearing masks now are experiencing a similar problem – they can't see the smile of greeting on someone's face behind the mask.

We were already paranoid about touching due to professional groups such as priests, therapists, and counselors touching in ways they shouldn't have. Business executives were committing sexual advances toward their staff. Hollywood has had more than its share of inappropriate contact. Now there's a pandemic and more paranoia.

Yes, precaution is necessary, but we don't want to throw away what we know is healthy for each of us. Healing, loving hugs from uninfected family members and friends should be given as much national strategic importance as the economy and our medical health system. It may be a long time before the routine of daily life begins to resemble the familiar pattern disrupted so quickly and dramatically over the past few months. Our need for healing human contact should not have to wait that long.

Here is my proposal: Everyone is to adopt the dual moniker of "giver of healing hugs" and "receiver of healing hugs." The special feature: Healing hugs can only be initiated by the receiver, and then the giver either can accept or refuse.

It starts with a statement from the hug receiver like, "I could use a healing hug right now." After the healing hug is received, the receiver gives thanks and positive feedback to encourage improved healing contact. Precautions such as gloves and masks are still important, but uninfected hugs can go a long way to helping reconnect families and friends.

Healing contact, when done with a sacred intent to promote well-being, can be a part of the healing relationship. Pandemic restrictions make it difficult to provide or receive healing contact. Right now, at the end of 30 self-imposed days of social isolation restricted to a small hotel room because we are between homes, and with minimal access to decent food, I really could use a big, healing hug. I know I am looking forward to saying to my grandchildren, "I need a healing hug."

Relationship Survival in Adversity

My wife and I left our New England home on April 4 and moved into a Midwest home on the 22nd – a total of 18 days in the dark, cramped quarters of various motel rooms. We have almost 50 years together and communication is one of our strong suits. But these 18 days were unusually difficult.

The experience of dealing with the pandemic restrictions is not unlike managing Parkinson's disease. The same principles are vital: sharing or asking for understanding and accommodation, making time and space for individual needs, and paying attention to communication.[149] One could surmise that our life with Parkinson's perhaps prepared us, in part, for the "new normal" imposed by the pandemic.

First, and probably not foremost in the minds of some, being confined to close quarters with your intimate partner tends to increase intimacy frequency. If you prepare for this, the experience can be more enjoyable. The usual diversions of life routines no longer distract. The need for intimacy may increase to help you connect with each other and express support and understanding. It can reinforce that the relationship is more accepting of the frailties of disease or aging, and therefore that the physical person is as important as the emotional or psychological person.

Second, more time must be given to communication. You might think that you have more access to knowing the other's needs because you are living in a confined space with your partner. Maybe that can happen when the world is not in pandemic chaos, or when Parkinson's progression hasn't created new chaos in our lives. Right now, though, so much emotion is swirling around because of the pandemic, which

---

[149] "7 Ways to Improve Communication in Relationships" by Birgit Ohlin, MA, BBA. Published on Positivepsychology.com, July 11, 2020.

easily leads to misunderstandings. We found ourselves making assumptions about the other's needs and then being wrong. Extended, close human proximity does not equate to more human understanding. That wisdom is found within a healing relationship, which is erratic and elusive during these apocalyptic times. The extra time spent by honestly and calmly asking and answering, "How are you doing?" will pay off rich dividends for the relationship.

Third, use phrases like "I feel" or "I need," rather than "you did" or "you don't" statements. Seems simple, but the louder the stress and chaos, the harder it is to do this. The accuracy of statements that express how you are feeling or what you need relies upon the accurate identification of emotion. Emotional intelligence is widely varied, but there is usually someone close to you who has a high EQ. It is often that person you know as a "good listener." There are also 1-800 helplines. In these times of social distancing, with short fuses everywhere, more precise descriptions of emotions are needed. It's not easy to stay in touch with feelings when there is a livid internal eruption happening every day. Practicing threshold management along with accurate and compassionate "I feel" statements made our 18 days a bit easier. Mistakes will happen. These are tough times. We had our quarrels, but we tried our best not to end the day angry at each other.

In addition, we divided the room in half – my space, your space. We also tried to have a normal daily schedule, despite how obviously abnormal the situation was. We set aside time where one partner supported the other for half the day. This routine included wellness activities. We had to be flexible with the half-day guideline because on some days one partner needed more time. We took turns throwing each other life preservers when the darkness began to engulf. We tried to be patient and support each other while also being open to asking for and receiving compassion.

Throughout the whole ordeal, we kept telling each other that we knew this move would be tough, but also brief, and that we didn't want 18 days to ruin 50 years of partnership. We continued to discover new possibilities that will be useful years from now, and we seek to continue as partners living with a chronic disease.

I've touched on several essays about relationship, each looking at different aspects. Even though I wrestle with the difficult symptoms of this chronic illness, I still make a concerted effort to minimize its interference in the relationship with my life partner, Mrs. Dr. C. The relationship essays seek to pass on this wisdom because a healthy relationship greatly benefits living well with Parkinson's disease.

Making the Connection

In *Talking to Strangers*, author Malcolm Gladwell[150] posits that we are lousy at knowing the intent of strangers. We have no better success than chance in determining whether someone is lying or telling the truth. One explanation why is called *truth default theory*.[151] Simply stated, when we meet strangers, we default to our beliefs about people in general. These beliefs shape how we interpret all the available cues gathered while talking to a stranger. This process of "sizing up" is how we arrive at our truth default position when talking to others, but the research suggests most of us, even those

---

[150] Gladwell, Malcolm. *Talking to Strangers: What We Should Know about the People We Don't Know*. Little, Brown & Co.; 1st edition (2019).
[151] Levine, Timothy R., Distinguished Professor & Chair of Communication Studies, University of Alabama at Birmingham. *Duped: Truth-Default Theory and the Social Science of Lying and Deception*. University of Alabama Press, 2019.

well-trained in human communication, are not particularly good at accurately reading people. Yet, experiencing that special connected feeling when meeting someone for the first time is the muse for poets, authors, and songwriters.

In my research on empathy, I looked at this problem of making an accurate connection that moves beyond the initial truth default position established by belief bias. I found that there is a certain type of relationship where the accuracy of sensing the other is improved over the truth default position. I call this the "healing relationship." Practicing healers, and those who have experienced healing with these healers, describe the healing relationship in sacred terms. The problem with science based on normative statistics, like the research on knowing if someone is lying, is that it gives you a snapshot of the general population while simultaneously discarding the outliers. Mystics and healers are often considered outliers of society. It would be interesting to see how they would fare in determining when someone is lying.

I describe empathy as having the following characteristics: reception, reflection, mutuality, proper intent, and developmental level. Within the healing relationship, the intent of empathy is solely to promote well-being of the other. It is a process of receiving sensory information about the other, reflecting that back accurately, and arriving at mutual understanding through this reception-reflection process. My ability to empathize is based on my skill in using empathy, which can be described as a developmental level.[152] Those who practice empathy at a high developmental level understand the concept differently than those who practice at the beginning level. While teaching graduate level counselors, I saw this often. Beginning counselors often refer to their truth default position when meeting patients for the first time,

---

[152] Chapter 1: The Nature of Empathy and Compassion, published on www.DrC.life

supporting the argument by Gladwell.

Despite how often we poorly read strangers, there is always the possibility that we can make a connection. There is the possibility that when we meet another person for the first time, we can let go of the truth default position and enter a meaningful healing relationship. We know we cannot do this with everyone. There just are some people with whom we cannot connect, and that is OK. What is exciting is that we are capable of a healing connection, setting aside our biases, deeply listening to another, and entering the compassion space, which opens the door to a shared human experience of healing.

There are two ways to look at the idea of a shared human experience. First is to look at shared context, two people witnessing the same thing, like the events of 9/11 or the assassination of JFK. The two people having witnessed the same event have a shared context and in that way a shared human experience. This does not mean that they feel or think about the event in the same way.

The second way to look at shared human experience is to identify empathy as a shared inner experience – two people sharing the feelings and sensations of the moment. Skilled empathy practitioners and the patients who have sat with them describe this shared inner experience process. The possibility of a healing connection exists even though we often misjudge reading people. Maybe the truth default position exists because we hope our talking with strangers will reveal the possibility of making a meaningful connection. It is this possibility that promotes growth and development of relationships, family, and society more than efforts to guard against the problems caused by the occasional liar.

For six years, I ran a compassion questionnaire on the Internet. There were two questions about the life-changing impact of relationships: one addressing the impact of a compassionate relationship, and the other addressing the impact of a harmful relationship. Of the approximately 600 respondents, over 90% rated the life impact of the compassionate relationship higher than the impact of the harmful relationship. The responses support the importance of the healing relationship, for not only experiencing the healing moment, but for our well-being over a lifetime. Making healthy connections makes our lives better. Knowing that a shared healing experience is possible makes living with a chronic disease like Parkinson's, even during stressful times, easier.

It's the Little Things

"Be one with the moment." Hogwash! I can't be one with the darkness. Yet, I do understand the power of the darkness for shaping my behaviors. I see the darkness as pure survival and protection against possible threats. It is a hyper-focus on self-survival along with unhealed battle wounds that constantly provide mortar for the walls of defense. There's little room for empathy and compassion. It is a good state of consciousness for a solo battle against threats of harm, but potentially damaging on personal relationships. Being consumed by darkness is an uncommon event in my life. However, being touched in little ways by the wounded warrior state of consciousness happens every day.

Every day, I have short emotional outbursts with frustration in connection with my Parkinson's decreased motor coordination and loss of vision abilities. Add to this chronic pain and surges of exaggerated emotion, and the result is that I work hard on calming my emotions dozens of times during the day. For the most part, I can self-contain these surges. Sometimes, I can't.

I was surprised – and I don't usually get surprised – at how small these inner outbursts are at the beginning. They only grow larger when left unattended, much like all the overgrown weeds in the unattended yard of our new home. Building a new sanctuary at the new home requires looking past the weeds, not getting overwhelmed with how much work there is, and being pleased with any progress. The same can be applied to personal healing work.

The journey taken to arrive at our new home was the hardest thing I have ever done. I became quite ill along the way. Not eating, not exercising, not socializing, and barely able to eke out weekly online columns. My body had trouble doing the simplest of things, such as going to the store with Mrs. Dr. C. for groceries. I am a mess. A serious health setback like this takes courage, patience, and support from friends and family to recover. The healing relationship provides a map. But that map is very fragile in the beginning stages of recovery. I made a promise to myself to find a way to heal, to do better, and to record the journey in these essays. If I can't walk it, I'm not going to talk it.

In the past, I was happy to keep big outbursts out of the home and out of important relationships. That has changed with the idea that the little inner emotional outbursts are equally challenging to manage. This was discovered while gardening. The soil here is very clay rich. I can grab a hunk and shape it into a baseball that keeps its shape when thrown. The soil also holds a lot of water. In addition, our new yard as a lot of trees. This combination of wet clay rich soil and lots of tree roots makes it difficult to put in new garden beds. I found myself struggling physically and swearing at both the clay soil and the roots. I don't think they heard me. They were still in the way of my next shovel thrust.

This may seem obvious, but the soil isn't trying to be annoying and the roots are not trying to get in my way. I chose to build the garden beds at this location for aesthetic reasons. This means I chose the location because I can see in my mind the vision of sanctuary that will surround my home when I am done. What I should say is, "Be happy for the opportunity." With every shovelful of wet heavy root-tangled mud, "This is going to look beautiful. Take a deep breath. Look at the garden and say, 'Thank you.'" I will fail. I will yell at the mud again. It is not about perfection: it is about improving quality of life. It is about opening the door to the possibility of more moments of well-being by attending to the little things that support the healing journey.

I have been applying this "little things practice." Breathing through (and calming down) within seconds of each tiny emotional surge. It helps make threshold management easier, resulting in more time and energy for enjoyable things. If I can manage the little things, and they come into my life from many more sources than gardening, I hope to do much better at managing the "big" ones.

Failed at Threshold Management and Paid the Price

"Yuck! It peed all over me," exclaimed my granddaughter as she released the toad back into the forest. "That's just his natural defense mechanism," replied her father. Like the toad, we too have our natural defense mechanisms. They are automatically called upon when a threat is perceived, real or not. The toad was not in any real harm, but the defense mechanisms reacted anyway. This happens with us too. Persistent threat exposure, real or not, over an extended time has negative consequences like crossing over the threshold of emotional control and having to pay the price.

Normally crossing the threshold of emotional control is a brief event: crying outburst, temper expression, and yelling eruption. But when there is persistent threat of harm over an extended time, threshold management becomes more difficult, the defense mechanisms are put in place more often, and the occurrences of crossing the threshold occur more often. Left unattended, this chronic defense against perceived threats, combined with regular loss of control, leads to what I call "darkness."

It is not easy for me to write about. First, I have only been immersed in darkness twice in my life and both times were following extended periods of threat to my well-being. Secondly, I have not delved into the published material on this topic. I do know that depression and anxiety are a challenge for nearly half of the people diagnosed with Parkinson's disease.[153] But the experience of darkness is not limited to people with such diagnoses. It can happen to anyone of us – patients or caretakers or family or friends – when exposed to persistent perceived threat over an extended time.

The darkness experience can be described as crossing over the threshold of emotional control and being stuck there. There is a flood of pain and wanting to do anything to escape that pain. Strong defense mechanisms are put in place to prevent any possibility of additional pain. The world gets closed off and a fragile ego is guarded night and day against insult. A simple phrase, such as, "Would you like to come over for a visit?" is interpreted as "I'm offended that you would even doubt that I would like to come and see you." There is spilling-out behavior, emotions leading to behaviors that are expelled onto others within the person's sphere of influence – like kicking the dog when you had a bad day. There is also a lot of "barking at the moon." I use that phrase for describing a stream of complaining directed at all those things wrong in

---

[153] Gallagher, David A. and Anette Schrag. "Psychosis, apathy, depression and anxiety in Parkinson's disease." *Neurobiology of Disease*, Volume 46, Issue 3, 2012, Pages 581-589, ISSN 0969-9961, https://doi.org/10.1016/j.nbd.2011.12.041.

the world, most of which I have little control over. Yet, I sit here in the darkness howling at all those things.

Another reason why it is hard for me to write about darkness is because I feel like a failure – an excessively big failure. When inside the darkness, I feel no compassion towards anyone, including myself. There is no faith, no serenity, no beauty, no meaning, and no purpose. It is very much the opposite of the authentic me that I choose to share with the world. Yet it was real, and I hated it. But as a writer, I chose to sit in the darkness and observe. I was surprised to see the intensity and severity of the defense mechanisms. These were 10-foot-thick concrete walls surrounding me, not letting anything in, but also not let anything out. I could see Mrs. Dr. C. trying to reach through the rock walls, bloodied knuckles to show for it. She never left my side.

One of the worst problems with the darkness experience is the lack of self-observation and accurate self-monitoring. It is one of the reasons why it is so hard to navigate solo.[154] Realistically sitting in the darkness is truly a horrible experience – a serpent coiled around my soul with fangs sunk deep, sucking out the light. I knew I was not thinking clearly and could not be in the darkness one second longer. I softly screamed, "I need help" with the deepest sincerity and open vulnerability that I could muster. Mrs. Dr. C. offered the sacred healing relationship and that pulled me back. It is almost impossible to navigate out of the darkness sailing solo.

---

[154] Yang, Sarah, et al. "Psychosocial Interventions for Depression and Anxiety in Parkinson's Disease." *Journal of Geriatric Psychiatry and Neurology*, vol. 25, no. 2, June 2012, pp. 113–121, doi:10.1177/0891988712445096.

She Has the Power:
Conversation with Neo

Neo exclaims, "That was amazing, Dr. C., that Mrs. Dr. C. applied the 'healing relationship' and 'poof!' you're all better!"

I grimaced at Neo's remark. It might sound that simple, but the process is much more involved. "Remember she has been with me for a long time. That is the special knowledge that Mrs. Dr. C. has. As James Taylor wrote in his song, *Something in the Way She Moves*, 'She has the power to go where no one else can find me, yes, and silently remind me, the happiness and the good times that I know, but as I had got to know them.' She is a witness to the best of me."

"You have mentioned the healing relationship in 12 essays," Neo points out. "I've read all that, but I still don't understand how it works."

I settle back for a comfortable position to explain to Neo the development of the concept. Sounding very professorial, I begin, "From the beginning of human community, healers, shamans, have been an important part of a sustainable social collective. Healers are often chosen by the tribe because of a 'gift' for sensing the inner person. They often undergo years of training, rites of passage, vision quests, or other initiations by the elder shaman. Some of these initiates pass from the ordinary to the extraordinary, and some do not. Those who do learn the intricate dance that is the healing process within the healing relationship. Only a few will become skilled healers knowing how to use the healing relationship."

During my soliloquy, I can make out Mrs. Dr. C. opening the door and coming in, laden down with groceries. I offer to help, and she asks, "What have you been up to while I was out?"

I mention Neo's amazement at the healing relationship. "It is his contention that all the stress was eliminated, and problems solved with your intervention and use of the healing relationship when I was in distress."

Turning back to Neo's attention, I explain, "I have mentioned in several essays that address the healing relationship to describe various parts. Here is a holistic experience connected to the phenomenon that cannot be known through a process that reduces it to singular events. Within this whole event is the possibility of experiencing a sacred, well-being moment. The possibility of a sacred well-being is available to everyone, trained and untrained, anytime, anywhere. Training with the healing relationship increases the probability it will occur but is not a guarantee. Training also helps with meaning-making."

Mrs. Dr. C. looks at me, adding, "What the 'good doctor' forgets is his brush with the darkness impacted both of us. We both had to go through that forest of emotions, despair, and fear. I think there are two more important points to make. One, I have never wanted to become a 'caretaker' instead of a 'wife.' Caretaker implies to me a distancing from the relationship of spouse. I feel if I take on that designation, it makes me emotionally separate. Second, I do not view the healing relationship as a cure. It does not change your symptoms of Parkinson's or the vision loss. It doesn't make them go away or stop you from having a change or progression or new conditions."

"That's really sad," Neo sighs. "So, what does the healing relationship do for you, Mrs. Dr. C.?"

She thinks for a moment, gazes out the window at the birds circling the feeders, and then says, "It gives me strength. It is a frightening thing for me to feel that there might be nothing I can do. I feel like I am helping to heal a wound, much like scar tissue over an injury. The Parkinson's and vision loss still happened, the pain is still there, and the scars will always be present. Neither of us can change that. But what we can do is hold on tight through the tough times. Sometimes, I can just be there to remind him that we can try to not put ourselves in situations where things get out of control."

Neo looks back to me for my reaction. I admit, "I know better. The healing relationship provides the map, and when I do not fully use it, I can expect a return to those difficult emotions. Using the healing relationship comes down to believing it is possible, and then having the experience and then learning how to use it."

Mrs. Dr. C. points at the shopping bags. "It would also help if you could put away some groceries with me."

Choosing What to do When Bad Things Happen

"I'm still not feeling well. I should go to the doctor." Mrs. Dr. C said with a pained look. I gave her a quick glance, and without even a hesitation in garden shoveling said, "OK. It's important that you attend to your health." She asked if I would like to go with her. I replied, "Not this time. I really want to get this part of the garden done today." The rest of the afternoon was consumed by this garden goal. I know she was disappointed.

I chose to direct all my attention and energies on this goal alone. I chose to ignore the little things that amplified my emotions one little moment at a time. I chose to ignore what I call my "little things practice." I watched as those unattended little moments gradually built up a crescendo. And yet, I chose to ignore the warnings maintaining attention on that precious garden goal. The consequences were felt in my personal relationship as emotional flooding became nearly unmanageable. I knew I had chosen an unhealthy path, yet it felt like I was powerless to choose any other. At the time, it seemed especially important to me that I complete the garden goal. Looking back, I can see that the failure to attend to the little things in favor of a singular goal orientation created negative consequences both personally and interpersonally.

Putting the little things practice in place is difficult under the best conditions, but it's much more challenging when bad things are happening –dealing with a chronic disease like Parkinson's, a partner with a chronic disease, a pandemic, and all the tasks that need to be fixed when settling into a new home in a new culture. Little things practice requires that I choose to focus my attention on the little things. Bad things can consume my resources, whether due to the energy needed for problem-solving or the energy used for coping. When the number of stressors and demands on my attention exceeds my available resources, I can get overwhelmed and end up at that precipice of threshold management. I can't engage my little things practice when approaching that precipice because the resources needed are being used elsewhere.

In a previous essay, I talked about brain therapy and training the conductor who oversees the "Grand Central Station" in our brains. Think of the conductor as the attention director. Sensory, memory, and emotional stimuli come into the "Grand Central Station." The conductor helps decide which stimuli are the most important and thus need to be granted quicker access and more attention. This is especially true when learning a new skill like little things practice. After some years of skill building, memory comes into play and it gets a bit easier. But in the beginning, it's like stepping off a four-lane highway and bushwhacking your way through the forest to carve out a new path. The new path of little skills practice is used to replace an old history of coping skills, much of which are no longer effective.

The brain is capable of growing new neurological connections, provided that the brain is not so damaged that the connections can no longer grow through that cerebral space. When that happens (and there are lots of ways to create damaged areas of the brain), then the challenge is to develop compensatory strategies that will support neurological connections growing around the damage – bushwhacking that new path through the forest. The conductor will need to be called upon to redirect attention to the new path, the path of little things practices – whether through or around. For me, it is much like putting in new gardens: it takes time, patience, persistence, and support. It will take years for the new gardens to take form as they have in previous homes. It will also be so with my progress on little things practice.

As I'm bushwhacking that new path of little things practice, I know I will fail. I will return to old habits, walking that easy four-lane highway instead of stumbling around in the forest. I must call upon the conductor continually throughout the day to direct the attention needed. Right now, in the early stages of my skill development, this is often draining. It is working. It is helping. But it is frustratingly slow!

Perhaps one of the most difficult aspects of brain training in the face of neurological trauma is that there is no quick, easy, fix. It takes hard work, concentrated effort, and continual practice over a long period of time. It is not easy for anyone. But patience with ourselves, and each other, helps us to succeed.

Begin the Journey

Hell on Earth, that's what it was: Shocked by becoming legally blind on top of worsening Parkinson's symptoms, including SEM attacks, chronic pain, and fatigue. People used to say, "You don't look like you have Parkinson's." But recent external and internal stressors have increased my symptoms.

At the same time, darkness consumed me. Made all the worse by a sedentary life and poor eating habits (sugar and fast foods), driven more by craving comfort than common sense. This is the state of ill health where my journey back to health begins. Tough starting point. At times, it feels impossible. But I have packed some things into a sacred backpack to make the journey easier.

It's not a heavy sacred backpack, as I have barely enough energy to motivate and move myself a few baby steps along the new health path, but it contains the essentials. The promise of the healing relationship not only showed me what the well-being experience is like, but gave me a map to find my way back. The wellness map has been expanded upon throughout the years, including the recent addition of little things practice. I also have the machete of the mystic scientist to help clear the weeds of confusion. The sacred backpack provides for all my material needs, so I can focus on the perils and wonders which lie ahead.

The path looks overwhelming, barely a gap between the trees where I can begin the journey. It starts with an unwavering commitment to starting. Not just any garden variety commitment, but a sacred commitment following the promises given with the healing relationship. Using the healing relationship, I know with certainty that viewing the healing journey as *sacred* will improve the possibility of a positive outcome. I make the sacred commitment to begin, and then, take the first little step.

Routine helps me take that first step. At the start of the healing journey, I focus on the three things which create the most distress on my physical system: a malfunctioning conductor, lack of exercise, and poor diet. The conductor training is a regular part of my daily routine now. I don't let my mind go out wandering alone anymore.

Routine is so helpful at the start of the journey back. Because it is "in my schedule" it becomes regular, routine, and anticipated. No thinking about it. I just do it. In this, I again discover my little things practice. The conductor training, exercise, and diet become sacred activities: mindful, deliberate, and revered.

Other writers speak to the importance of exercise for people who have a chronic illness, especially Parkinson's. Those starting physical activities with Parkinson's always encounter motor hesitation. I find it helpful to engage in a form of exercise which I enjoy – gardening. I look forward to getting outdoors in the greenspace and the work on creating a new sacred sanctuary. Lots of opportunities for little things practice.

Diet has been a topic I have avoided because it is outside my scope of expertise. The literature about its influence on the probability of positive outcomes for those with Parkinson's is often contradictory and confusing. For example: Eating chocolate might be beneficial, but consuming sugar is more habit than nutritional necessity.[155] Returning to my favorite scientific diet research *The China Study*,[156] I am again certain that eliminating sugar and high-fat content meals will increase the possibility of a positive health outcome. Sugar is the first to go – but gradually, over a six-month period. It's not about perfection, but rather about slowly making the switch from sugar treats to fruit treats, fresh fruit, and protein supplements. There is an addictive quality to sugar.

---

[155] Naughton, Paul, Mary McCarthy, and Sinéad McCarthy. "Acting to self-regulate unhealthy eating habits. An investigation into the effects of habit, hedonic hunger and self-regulation on sugar consumption from confectionery foods." *Food Quality and Preference*, Volume 46, 2015, Pages 173-183, ISSN 0950-3293, https://doi.org/10.1016/j.foodqual.2015.08.001.

[156] Campbell, T. Colin and Campbell, Thomas M. II. *The China Study: Revised and Expanded Edition: The Most Comprehensive Study of Nutrition Ever Conducted and the Startling Implications for Diet, Weight Loss, and Long-Term Health*. Ben Bella Books; Revised edition 2016.

Decreasing its consumption includes dealing with cravings. I don't fight with it. Instead, I recreate in my mind the physical memories of being sick when I consume too much sugar. Holding onto that thought, I confront my cravings and say, "15 minutes of feeling good is not worth 15 hours of suffering."

The journey back to health has begun, with three little steps: conductor training, exercise, and healthy diet. It is framed as a sacred process, like a sacred tea ceremony using my wellness map. Not only have I discovered many more opportunities for little things practice, but in doing so, I have discovered an everyday calmness. Not like the bliss moment of being caressed in calmness. Instead, it is a soft gentle cooling breeze that is present for multiple days. Sounds impossible, given where I started. Amazing! Feels like I have a protective shield now.

Crack in the Shield: Conversation with Neo

Sirens, flashing red and blue hazard lights, and Dr. C. slumped in a gray felt recliner with the pallor to match. A greatly worried Neo exclaims, "What is going on here?"

Mrs. Dr. C. pokes her head out from around the kitchen. "It was a real rough night here, wasn't it?" Dr. C. nods his head and waves his hand to signal her to continue the conversation without him. "The carbon monoxide alarm went off and we called 911. They found the problem – a faulty water heater. The fire department cleared out the bad air and disabled the unit. But Dr. C. had already had too much exposure to a toxic situation. I guess there is a crack in that new wellness shield."

"I know Doc was really excited about his wellness shield, but it looks like it doesn't work." Neo looks at Dr. C., who resembles something from *The Walking Dead*. "He really looks terrible."

Mrs. Dr. C. calmly replies, "He's been working on rehabilitative programs to help people with chronic illness like Parkinson's disease for several years now. But it is not a magical shield to protect against highly toxic situations.

He has been through a lot of physical, emotional, and psychological stress recently and is in a fragile place in the recovery process. Exposure to toxic or intensely stressful situations can overwhelm him. Then all his PD symptoms flare up at the same time. It is just a big ugly mess. It's not the rehabilitation program for every day that failed. It was the additional exposure to something we did not anticipate."

"But don't we all have protective measures we think will guard us against harm?" Neo inquires.

"We all have ways to incorporate lifestyle changes into our routines or wellness maps. If these steps are applied in a very mindful way, they can help. Unfortunately, there are situations or external causes that just exacerbate the Parkinson's symptoms. Dr. C. has always exhibited a sensitivity to detergent chemicals. He was given a sensitivity test to determine his reactions and ranked among the highest score of the 'hypersensitive individual.'

"It took years for the VA to conduct multiple studies to link Agent Orange used in Vietnam combat missions[157] for disability claims. They did a study in the Camp LeJeune

---

[157] The Health and Medicine Division (formally known as the Institute of Medicine) of the National Academy of Sciences, Engineering, and Medicine concluded in its report "Veterans and Agent Orange: Update 2008" released July 24, 2009, that there is "suggestive but limited evidence that exposure to Agent Orange and other herbicides used during the Vietnam War is associated with an increased chance of developing Parkinson's disease." As a result, VA recognized Parkinson's disease as associated with exposure to Agent Orange or other herbicides during military service. VA's final regulation recognizing this association took effect on October 30, 2010.

training camp and discovered that toxins in the water[158] resulted in increase in development of eight different medical conditions, including Parkinson's." Mrs. Dr. C. continues, "Dr. C was exposed to both. We are thankful that the Veterans Administration has stepped up to address the disability of Veterans from these toxic exposures. But other chemical exposures possibly resulting in disease development have been discovered from the use of more common products like weed control.[159] So, we try to avoid those products. Even

---

[158] The new federal rule that there was "sufficient scientific and medical evidence" to establish a connection between exposure to the contaminated water and eight medical conditions for purposes of awarding disability compensation covers active duty, Reserve and National Guard members who developed one of eight diseases: adult leukemia, aplastic anemia, bladder cancer, kidney cancer, liver cancer, multiple myeloma, non-Hodgkin's lymphoma, and Parkinson's disease. Documents uncovered by Veterans groups over the years suggest Marine leaders were slow to respond when tests first found evidence of contaminated ground water at Camp Lejeune in the early 1980s. Some drinking water wells were closed in 1984 and 1985, after further testing confirmed contamination from leaking fuel tanks and an off-base dry cleaner. The Marine Corps has said the contamination was unintentional, occurring when federal law didn't limit toxins in drinking water. The 246-square-mile military training complex was established in 1941. The new federal rule covers Camp Lejeune and Marine Corps Air Station New River, including satellite camps and housing areas. Reported on *PBS NewsHour in Nation*, by Hope Yen, Associated Press, on January 13, 2017.
[159] Glyphosate is by far the most widely used herbicide in the United States, and probably worldwide. It is used on nearly every acre of corn, cotton, and soybeans grown in the US. You may have sprayed it on your lawn or garden. But many jurisdictions, in more than two dozen countries, have banned or restricted its use. Among the latest: Los Angeles County announced last month that it was suspending use of glyphosate on county property until more is known about its health effects. Bayer says on its website that the weed killer has been thoroughly tested, and "an extensive body of research" shows that products containing it "can be used safely and that glyphosate is not carcinogenic." Cynthia Curl, an environmental health scientist at Boise State University in Idaho who studies the chemical, said, "many assumptions have been

something as innocuous as talcum powder has been identified as a potential carcinogen."[160]

Mrs. Dr. C. pauses. "I can't help but wonder if Dr. C. is more susceptible to chemical hazards. I felt fine and did not show any symptoms from our recent exposure. Dr. C. looked and acted like he had been hit by a ton of bricks. We try to keep ourselves safe, but situations are going to come up unexpectedly and we can't always predict or rely on past experiences to know when something is going to adversely affect him. While many chemical exposures do not necessarily cause Parkinson's, we have to be vigilant about the ones that exacerbate his symptoms – the ones that slip through the crack in the shield."[161]

---

made about the safety of glyphosate that are now being actively questioned. We will see an explosion of information about glyphosate, and it's about time. We're really playing catch-up on this one." Reported on *PBS Newshour*, by Marla Cone, Kaiser Health News, April 8, 2019.

[160] It is not clear if consumer products containing talcum powder increase cancer risk. Studies of personal use of talcum powder have had mixed results, although there is some suggestion of a possible increase in ovarian cancer risk. There is very little evidence at this time that any other forms of cancer are linked with consumer use of talcum powder. Until more information is available, people concerned about using talcum powder may want to avoid or limit their use of consumer products that contain it. Written by The American Cancer Society medical and editorial content team, February 4, 2020.

[161] A new research report contributes to the increasing evidence that repeated occupational exposure to certain chemical solvents raises the risk for Parkinson's disease. Of the six chemicals investigated, researchers concluded that two common chemical solvents, trichloroethylene (TCE) and perchloroethylene (PERC), are significantly linked to development of this disease. PERC is the leading chemical used in garment dry cleaning. TCE is the most frequently reported organic groundwater contaminant, was once used as general anesthetic and coffee decaffeinating agent, and is still used widely as a metal degreasing agent. TCE has also been linked to Parkinson's by other research groups. Researchers at the University of Kentucky, Lexington, and the Kangwon National University in South Korea have reported an association between

Neo says, "That makes sense. Is Dr. C. going to be OK?"

Dr. C. clears his voice. Neo and Mrs. Dr. C. look in his direction as he begins to talk. "The best program for improving well-being is one that is tailored specifically to the one individual seeking help. My personal program came with instructions on how to implement it. But life sort of took a turn I didn't expect." Dr. C. gives Mrs. Dr. C. a hug and says, "The biggest lesson here – I am looking forward to getting back on track."

Rethinking Exercise

I hate facing the effort it takes to start daily exercise. I hate the way I feel the next day – like I have been pummeled with nunchuks. But ever since my Marine Corps training, I have enjoyed the benefits of exercise. I know it is hard to get up and engage in physical activity. This is particularly true when facing the motor hesitation of Parkinson's. It is hard to exercise facing the level of discomfort that is going to follow – the post-exercise stiffness is compounded by the rigidity associated with Parkinson's. Yet, despite these difficulties, the benefits of exercise far exceed the temporary increase in discomfort.

Starting exercise after being sedentary combined with neuromuscular malfunctions requires special considerations. The Marine Corps boot camp approach just is not going to work. Last time I tried that, I ended up with multiple muscle

---

TCE and Parkinson's in highly exposed industrial workers and have also demonstrated that TCE causes neurodegeneration in animal models. This study, supported in part by the National Institute of Neurological Disorders and Stroke (NINDS), a part of the National Institutes of Health, appears in the Nov. 14, 2011 issue of Annals of Neurology and reported by the Institutes of Health, *News Release*, November 14, 2011.

injuries. A new approach to exercise came from three ideas: mindful movements, little things practice, and long movements adapted from LSVT exercise recommendations.

In the study, "Effect of Exercise on Motor and Nonmotor Symptoms of Parkinson's Disease," the authors report "LSVT BIG therapy is designed to overcome amplitude deficits associated with PD. This therapy improves proprioception[162] through increasing amplitude together with sustained attention and cognitive involvement by mentally focusing on individual movements."[163] In other words, I am concentrating on where my body is, what it is doing, and paying attention by focusing on the task at hand.

My new exercise program incorporates activities that focus on movements that are long and slow while simultaneously engaged in a mindful focus on the little things. This new exercise program is also tied to something that will continually motivate me to move past the PD hesitation to start. I discovered, in some ways rediscovered, the answer with landscape gardening.

What is great about landscape gardening is that there are so many different types of motor tasks that need to be accomplished: shoveling, hauling with wheelbarrow, planting, raking, clipping, and pruning. Knowing that I need more light physical activity, for both warming up and for bad days, where I can only put in short durations, I am installing a white gravel Zen path. The small gravel pieces, less than an inch in diameter, are incredibly easy to rake with long mindful movements. Light and easy warm-up exercise has become mandatory for me before any physical activity.

The one day I forgot resulted in strained muscles that

---

[162] Perception or awareness of the position and movement of the body.
[163] Dashtipour, Khashayar et al. "Effect of exercise on motor and nonmotor symptoms of Parkinson's disease." *Parkinson's disease* vol. 2015 (2015): 586378. doi:10.1155/2015/586378

required too much time to heal. The good thing is I now know what strained muscle pain feels like and how it is different from Parkinson's muscle pain and different from post-exercise pain. I now know why the light warm-up exercise in a mindful state needs to happen before I tackle the larger landscape gardening projects.

Getting back into exercise after being sedentary for so long requires patience – lots and lots of patience. I see so many things in my vision for our yard. But I know if I push myself in that old boot camp way, I am going to end up injured and not able to accomplish my vision. But patience means slowing down, and slowing down feels like I am not accomplishing "great" things. If I think I am not accomplishing, then I am not successful, and if I cannot be successful, then I feel no need for starting at all. It is a devious cycle that ignores the practice of "little things" and becomes a reason to not exercise. Mindful, light motor exercise activities break that cycle. Like Tai Chi and yoga, the long mindful movements help me motivate out of sedentary life and into a balanced exercise regime.

Gardening is also good for the mind, and what is good for the mind is good for the body. My approach to gardening is different now. My first impression of the change is that my actions are calmer, framed in sacred intent. But, in all honesty, I am still sorting all that out. Using this new approach to exercise, while being creative with landscape gardening, is making positive changes in my health.

There are many obstacles created by the Parkinson's disease that can make engaging in exercise a difficult process. I find the more I understand those obstacles, the better I am at finding my way around them. The bottom line – find a way to exercise that you enjoy, that you can access readily, and then stay motivated and engaged.

A Fresh Look at Chronic Pain

For fifteen years, I have been a failure at managing my chronic pain. Initially, I was prescribed oxycodone and gabapentin for the pain. I wasn't happy being prescribed the oxycodone but it was the only treatment offered by my provider at that time. After the PD diagnosis, I was put on levodopa, which decreased my pain to the point where oxycodone was no longer needed. I also tried alcohol in another provider-prescribed attempt to make the pain vanish. It felt more like I was replacing it with "feel-goods." I know chasing after "feel-goods" is not the right approach for me, so I stopped all the pain medications and the prescribed "glass of wine at night" therapy except levodopa.

At this juncture, I wish to be truly clear that I am *not* recommending anyone stop their medications. This is my personal journey and decisions made with the consultation of my providers. For me, the risk of the opioid treatment far outweighed the benefits. Gabapentin in my system dulled my brain to the point where my cognitive abilities (or lack thereof) adversely affected my quality of life. It has only been within the last few months that all the pieces finally fell into place, revealing a new fresh approach to chronic pain management.

Chronic pain management is not just about popping a pill and hoping to be pain free. No matter what I do, I will always have PD chronic pain every day. The goal is to live better. Medications that seek to disguise this reality within the gawdy attire of society's "feel good" addictions always send up big red warning flags for me. The brain has a remarkable ability to rewire itself so that it can function better even with chronic pain. If I am putting chemicals in my brain, or a set of addictive thoughts/feelings, which interfere in my rehabilitative rewiring, then I must make a change or give up. Giving up and showing up are just a breath and a step a part.

The PD chronic pain management program I use incorporates many of these small changes to help me live better. Here is my list:

- Know your pain and identify the starting point clearly
- Exercise three to four times per week in a way that fits your abilities
- Take charge of personal well-being by developing a wellness map
- Use emotion threshold management
- Reduce toxic stress from all sources, including diet and environment
- Use medications to assist with (not replace) brain rewiring
- Draw upon your support system (including the sacred) to help with the rehab

This list reflects some of the information available on chronic pain management. Each small change supports a small increase in the space between chronic pain and the thought/feeling reaction to that pain. Each small change strengthens the stability of the pause. With a long enough pause, it is possible to call on the conductor who can then reroute the brain's response to pain and SEM attacks. Once the conductor is called upon, one can discover something more. One can discover a fresh new look at chronic pain management.

The old ways of coping with the pain were not working because the SEM attacks were causing an exaggeration of the pain signal and exaggerated emotions in me. In my search to live better with this, I discovered a new exercise approach – and along the way, a few gems of wisdom:

- Intense emotional experiences can exacerbate chronic pain
- Uncontrolled actions connected to intense emotional experiences can also increase pain

- Skilled meditators experience intense motions differently than the average person
- People with highly skilled conductors will experience intense emotion differently; seeing the intense emotional experiences, along with pain, from the viewpoint of the conductor, is not the same as the original emotional/pain experience

With patience and perseverance, I sat at the conductor's viewing window every day over four months. Many of the discoveries from this view are chronicled in my essays. In connection to SEM attacks is the idea of anxiety/sad emotion surges occurring without being tied to context. Many of the emotional surges were purely abnormal PD biochemicals with no environmental or conscious antecedent – just a surge of emotion due to brain chemistry. Given this to be true, and my history using a well-trained conductor, I passionately believed a new brain path would be found. At the time, I was just using the conductor's window to find a way to tone down the SEM attacks. What I discovered was a lot more and yet so simple:

The need to fight, to flee, or to act in a way to seek nurturing is an automatic, often instinctual, response to pain signals. If those pain signals are exaggerated, so can be the response. In my case, it is all based on illusion caused by an organic malfunction. There is no external threat which requires a fight/flight/nurture seeking response.

This perception of the difference between a thought/feeling and an observed thought/feeling isn't just an idea for me but rather an experienced phenomenon connected to the vision of a better life. At the conductor's window, I sat and watched the exaggerated illusionary signal, I watched the pain and emotions approach, and I saw them redirected down a new track leaving no consequence visible to others. I felt no fanfare, no bliss, no awe. Just a soft everyday calmness and a sense that I can do this conductor rerouting. In a prominent place in our home, I put up a calendar to document success. At the end of each day, I shared with Mrs. Dr. C. the placing of a big red checkmark for every day the conductor successfully reroutes the reaction to pain and the SEM attacks. It gave me a sense of accomplishment and a way for Mrs. Dr. C. to see how I was doing.

Tips for Dealing with Chronic Pain: A Review

My essays about pain and chronic pain have fallen a bit short. Here are some more commonsense tips that I use when medically appropriate.

Tip 1: I exercise. It may seem counterintuitive that working malfunctioning muscles will help the chronic pain, prevent falls (when combined with mindful movements), and improve quality of life. Core body strength will offset the muscle weakness and coordination issues. There are so many options available for finding the exercise program that motivates one to not stop. My choice is gardening as it combines the health benefits of nature and the ability to vary the type of motor task.

Tip 2: Decreasing stress is my second most important tip. Stress increases my physical symptoms. It diminishes my mental and psychological well-being. Stress is often tied to self-imposed demands on one's time and reservoir of energy. I don't have to give up on my dreams, just modify them – several times – to fit the disease.

Tip 3: I try to avoid toxic situations. Seeking sanctuary is not escaping the realities of life. It is giving me a chance to take a deep breath, evaluate, and control my reactions. Life is not perfect, but it can be worse by entering avoidable toxic situations or interactions that I know will be emotionally or psychologically stressful.

Tip 4: Dangerous chemicals that are not medically

prescribed – like caffeine, nicotine, and food allergies – add stress. Medication management is between you and your providers. I'm not afraid to speak up and let providers know that a medication isn't working. My brain is the best tool I have when used wisely.

Tip 5: Stay out of the high heat and hydrate. I have problems regulating my body temperature and need to monitor water intake. I can't rely only on *feeling* thirsty. The PD brain signals malfunction, and I don't have the physical signals telling me to get fluids.

Tip 6: Maintain a healthy weight. I have lost 30 pounds and it does reduce my chronic pain. Exercising becomes easier. With less strain on our bodies, we function better.

Tip 7: Don't hold back on bathroom visits. Seems like an unusual tip, but holding it in and delaying the bathroom visit puts extra stress on the muscles. These same muscles relieve the body of waste. If they are stressed, there can be increased pain. I can end up in the bathroom for hours afterwards. Non-motor problems, like constipation or diarrhea, or urinary and kidney problems, are well documented in PD.[164] I map out accessible bathrooms when traveling away from home.

Tip 8: Modify as needed any activity which increases body rigidity. For me, this includes negative emotions, sitting too long without moving, post-exercise stiffness, sleeping and, unfortunately, orgasms. I am using a mindful approach to decrease the pain associated with rigidity.[165]

Tip 9: I practice threshold management to keep emotions balanced. I don't have to be an emotional zombie, but runaway emotions can adversely impact me and others around me.

---

[164] Sakakibara, Ryuji, et al. "Bladder, bowel, and sexual dysfunction in Parkinson's disease." *Parkinson's disease* vol. 2011 (2011): 924605. doi:10.4061/2011/924605

[165] "43 People Comment on The Benefits of Mindfulness." Katie Holmes, published on Community Discussions, *Outwit Trade*, September 21, 2020.

Tip 10: Whenever possible, I try to be grateful, compassionate, and kind to myself with self-talk and live with a lightness of being. Another BioNews columnist wrote about "self-talk" and not identifying oneself as "suffering" from a disease.[166] That is a better alternative for me – to acknowledge its existence but not be defined by it.

Sleep and rest are crucial to my well-being and is a top ten tip. I've said before, "If I can't walk it, I won't talk it." I still wrestle with sleep issues. I know intimately that deficit rest or sleep will increase the pain. As the pain goes up, rest and sleep become more difficult. It is a repetitive loop which I have struggled with for more than a decade. The only tip I have found helpful is to take 10- to 15-minute muscle stretch breaks every two or three hours – even during sleep time. I can get six or seven hours of rest if I do this.

It is also important to embrace my support network. Mrs. Dr. C. and I communicate multiple times a day using a simple scale in response to, "How are you doing?" The scalar response is as follows: "I'm doing good," "Medium," "So-so," "Bad," or "Terrible day." Sometimes, Mrs. Dr. C. and I face "CHRONDI Forcing" where PD and chronic pain force me to disengage from any type of motor activity. Using this scale in my communication informs my family when the daily routine needs adjusting.

Let's Face It – Mindful Mouth Movements

Bit my tongue hard enough to draw blood, releasing that unique rusty-iron taste. This wasn't the first time. When I had teeth removed earlier in my life, leaving open spaces for a few weeks while artificial teeth were being made, my mouth muscles had difficulty adjusting. The consequences are quite

---

[166] "We Are What We Tell Ourselves." Jessie Ace, "Disabled to Enabled," published on Multiple Sclerosis News Today, May 26, 2020.

painful. The solution is mindful mouth movements.

Eating (particularly chewing) is like walking. It's an overlearned motor sequence we repeat without much thought. Most people can walk and chew gum at the same time. Just not me. I must direct mindful attention to both walking and chewing. When I do, there are few problems. When I don't, there are always negative consequences. It's another example of broken scenario looping.

It is not just chewing. I need to be mindful of swallowing. I can't be talking around the family dining table while I'm eating – not even between swallows. Mrs. Dr. C. dislikes the choking spasms that are the consequence. It can be scary for loved ones watching. I need to assign to the mouth one motor task at a time and pay attention.

Aspiration during drinking has been alleviated a bit by using a straw. I have a big cup with a screw-on top. It saves me from having to refill a small glass multiple times during the day. The top helps when I invariably miss reaching for it, potentially spilling the contents. The big cup requires a long straw. Strange enough, they are hard to find. Those drink straws from fast-food places don't extend much beyond the top edge of the cup. A little Internet searching, and we were able to find 14-inch straws. Another accommodation in the quest to manage PD.

Public speaking is something I enjoy doing and I dread the days when the PD thief arrives. I used to talk daily with other gamers inside a virtual reality computer game. But then the vision loss happened. Mrs. Dr. C. helps with my talking. She has profound hearing loss, so I need to increase my volume to almost a shout and do this without sounding angry. This gives me lots of vocal projection practice.

I find I need to slow down the speed of my words and make sure I can devote full attention to what I'm saying. I can't be emotionally distracted or engaged in thinking about things or occupied with the weekly "honey-do" list. All my attention is on speaking clearly, loudly, and calmly. I am worried that this is not enough mouth therapy to keep the old professorial voice in shape. I hope to return to playing the guitar and singing.

There seem to be conflicting reports of the influence of levodopa on swallowing and other related mouth movements like dysphagia.[167] Just recently, I have started clenching my teeth at night, confirmed by the dentist as nocturnal bruxism. Nocturnal bruxism is defined as "nighttime tooth clenching or grinding". Like many of the movement behaviors in PD, nocturnal bruxism is an involuntary behavior and not simply the result of stress. It's considered both a symptom of PD and a free-standing sleep disorder. Parkinson's Net writers further identify that,

> It's interesting to note that, while bruxism can happen at any time of day, <u>daytime versions are seldom a complaint in someone with PD</u>. Complaints of morning jaw pain, or the discovery of loosened or even broken teeth, may signal a case of nocturnal bruxism. Tight or sore neck muscles are also common. It might be easy to blame the pillow or aging for these problems, but it would be better to rule out bruxism first, as it can be treated.[168]

A study in the *Journal of Oral Rehabilitation* (2018)[169] states, "Patients with PD/PR[170] reported significantly more often bruxism during sleep and wakefulness than controls.

---

[167] Menezes C., Melo A. "Does levodopa improve swallowing dysfunction in Parkinson's disease patients?" *J Clin Pharm Ther*. 2009 Dec;34(6):673-6. doi: 10.1111/j.1365-2710.2009.01031.x. PMID: 20175800.

[168] "A Surprising Reason to See the Dentist: Oral Hygiene & Parkinson's." TK Sellman, published on Parkinson'sDisease.net, October 3, 2019. https://parkinsonsdisease.net/living/oral-hygiene-dentist/

[169] Verhoeff M.C., Lobbezoo F., Wetselaar P., Aarab G., Koutris M. "Parkinson's disease, temporomandibular disorders and bruxism: A pilot study." *J Oral Rehabil*. 2018 Nov;45(11):854-863. doi: 10.1111/joor.12697. Epub 2018 Aug 13. PMID: 30024048.

[170] PD is identified in the article as Parkinson's Disease; PR is referring to Parkinsonism, which is a general term of characteristic symptoms of PD.

Also, patients with PD/PR had more often possible TMD and reported a significantly higher mean pain intensity in the orofacial region than controls."

Neurologists generally do not screen for bruxism as a motor dystonia[171] and many dentists are not trained in recognizing the impact of PD on dental problems. A review of the literature indicates that only since 2015 has there been an increase in awareness of bruxism as a definable PD symptom. Instead, I work on paying attention to coordinating mind and mouth movements: daytime, nighttime, and all the time.

A Fresh Look at Depression and Chronic Illness

> When everything was at its worst,
> the darkness engulfed me.
> I yell out, "I hate my life."

In 2017, an estimated 7.1% of all US adults were diagnosed with depression at some point in their lives.[172] It is much worse for those with a chronic disease; up to 50% for those with Parkinson's experience depression.[173] This means many people with PD who also battle depression are people who did not have noticeable signs of depression before the chronic illness. I am one of those people.

Depression and chronic illness are intertwined. There is

---

[171] "Bruxism in the Neurology Clinic" by Martin Taylor, DO, PhD. Published on PracticalNeurology.com, September 2015.
[172] National Institutes of Mental Health. Mental Health Information, Statistics, Major Depression. 2019.
[173] Parkinson's Foundation. "Understanding Parkinson's: Non-Movement Symptoms, Depression." Reviewed by Dr. Chauncey Spears, Movement Disorders Fellow at the University of Florida, a Parkinson's Foundation Center of Excellence, undated.

grief connected to the losses caused by the disease. There is the feeling that no one can understand the intense suffering I endure. Then there is the pain – every day, unrelenting. Add life stressors (such as moving across country in the middle of a pandemic, and unhealthy habits in response to the stress) and the result is a compost pile fertile with seeds for depression.

To slow the development of depression, I have tried to change my reactions to the triggers. Life is quiet in our new home. Work on the new garden sanctuary is proceeding nicely. I developed a new way of looking at my chronic disease, thus decreasing the grief. Reaching out and connecting to others has soothed the loneliness. Regular exercise and pain management manage overall pain.

After these triggers of depression were tamed, I discovered two things: First, there is the physical appearance of depression due to the emotional contortions imparted by the disease. Second, there is a brain stimulus abnormality that creates surges of exaggerated emotion. Both contributed to my falling into the darkness. When I looked in the mirror I saw a stooped, old guy, head down, not smiling, not engaging, and grumpy. Here was a depressed man. The exaggerated emotion of frequent sadness festered in the new caricature.

Once I got out of the darkness and back into exercise with healthier habits (such as meditation), I began to question the utility of sadness. Meditation for me is like standing in a pond. At first, it's a raging storm, waves lapping up against my legs, fierce wind everywhere, dark clouds, thunder, lightning. There are a lot of signals coming into the brain from many different places so it's hard to meditate. Acceptance of my map to well-being, healthy living, and practicing mindfulness are all helpful.

Standing in the stormy pond, I can watch calmly as the storm passes through me. The surface of the pond becomes as still as polished mirror. It only lasts a few seconds before I have thrown the proverbial pebble. Last time I was there, I felt the ripples before the storm, a tickle against the skin on my legs. I looked up and felt a gentle breeze on my cheek. I realized the ripples were driven by the breeze. Then I heard a faint cry in that breeze. We are born helpless and instinctually cry out when in pain or when our survival needs aren't being met. The exaggerated surges of sadness are tied to this instinctual need to be nurtured.

There is nothing wrong with wanting a little nurturing. I've advocated for healing hugs. The problem comes when I let sadness run rampant in my brain – unrestrained, contaminating everything. It leads quickly to frequent sadness, then to overwhelming sadness. I get angry at feeling so sad. Soon, I'm spinning around in a dark place and I can't find the door. Feeling hopeless, I say, "I hate my life." I know the term "darkness" may have religious connotations, but I am not using it that way. Think of it more as a brain darkness. The brain is so focused on fight/flight and nurture-seeking that it cannot see anything else. One is blinded to all other forms of perception that could be generated by other regions of the brain. In hindsight, I felt blinded. Unfortunately, when in that darkness, I am convinced of my own point of view. It is difficult to navigate well.

Reframing depression as instinctual brain signals designed originally to enhance our survival radically changed my outlook. I clearly see the need to be nurtured is often not connected to anything that anyone can do to change the situation. Asking other people to address my need for nurturing, when there's nothing that they can do, is ignorant and possibly harmful.

I tore up that depressed old guy caricature. I cut my hair and my beard and I'm exercising my mouth into a smile more often. There is a new guy in town.

Putting Your Best Face Forward

The image of PD that I called a caricature in my essay on depression does not match how I see the illness and does not match what most people experience. We need a new face for the disease, one that reflects how people experience the illness and one that offers possibility instead of a prognostication of doom.

Researchers M.J. Armstrong and M.S. Okun, in their article entitled, "Time for a New Image of Parkinson Disease"[174] state, "People with Parkinson disease are living for many years without the profound disability." Most people who have the disease don't look like the classic image first identified by Sir William Richard Gowers in 1886. His description of an aged, frail, trembling man has been carried through the decades. This classic PD image introduces bias that affects inaccurate diagnoses, missed diagnosis (particularly in women), and contributes to the disease being invisible until it fits that classic image.

With this classic image comes a view that it has to all end badly, that the possibilities for a quality life are severely limited. It's a tough box to climb out of. A new face on PD needs to be inserted into education given to medical professionals. This new approach could cut down on misdiagnoses prior to receiving the PD diagnosis.[175]

Armstrong and Okun, authors of this important article, talk of a stigma attached to the classic PD image, a bias that shapes the mind into making a box into which all things PD

[174] Armstrong, M.J., Okun M.S. "Time for a New Image of Parkinson Disease." *JAMA Neurol.* Published online July 27, 2020. doi:10.1001/jamaneurol.2020.2412

[175] "Poll Finds 1 in 4 People with Parkinson Disease Misdiagnosed." Matthew Gavidia, *The American Journal of Managed Care*, published January 8, 2020. First reported in *The Guardian* from a poll conducted for the charity Parkinson's UK, December 2019.

must go. The classic image comes with a mental frame about what may occur, what can be a lurking shadow of fears surrounding PD. This bias may even extend into how we think about helping people who have been diagnosed with PD, including how we help ourselves. The authors of the article claim the classical image of PD can be a self-fulfilling prophecy and, in that way, impede well-being.

I have redesigned the image reflecting my chronic illness. I needed a new face for my illness. I don't have to wear that old image just because the medical profession thinks it's what the illness must look like. Trust me when I say I have struggled with that old image. One neurologist I saw suggested that I stop my medications so he could see signs of that old image. I have wanted to display that caricature just so my "invisible" illness would be seen. Maybe then my suffering would be understood. It felt like an injustice that I had to harm myself to meet the illusions of society. I couldn't wear it anymore.

The new face I use is the best face I can find – one that fits the science and is filled with possibility. I frame the chronic illness as a brain injury and open to brain healing simultaneously. The brain is responsible for both the illness and how we deal with it, including a sacred healing process. It includes the wellness map and all the tips for a quality of life included in my writing. That's my best face going forward.

I don't believe in that old caricature of PD. I think it contributes to being ill and limits possibilities. I believe in the power of the human brain to mold itself around an injury to function better despite the insult. The brain can change in response to what we ask it to do. We can think, act, and feel in a way that provides correct stimulation of the pathways necessary for building a bridge over the damaged area.

This is a model I used in my clinical career to help others suffering from a brain insult. Now I am applying that model to my own life and sharing the insights with my readers. I am pleased with the discoveries, like the role of the "conductor" that resulted from wearing this new face. It's nice not to be that "old, decrepit, depressed guy."

The overall focus of this book is to provide a fresh look at Parkinson's disease, to put a new face on it. It's my goal to discuss why I think this is possible.

It's my new face for going forward.

Overwhelmed and Not Moving: Conversation with Neo

Looking frantic, Neo sighs, "I can't handle all of this. Tips on how to live better with a chronic disease, tips on managing chronic pain, tips on depression, and putting on a new face. I get overwhelmed just thinking about it all. I want to be healthier, but I'm worried that I am not capable and won't get it right. It gets so that I am spinning in my head with so many thoughts and feelings and not moving. Before I know it, the day has slipped by and I am back to the same routine. I have little relief the next day from feeling miserable. It never changes."

Neo collapses in his neural chair. Dr. C. reaches out to Neo and says, "You saw the terrible state I was in after what happened. At times, it felt impossible to move. I woke every morning feeling miserable. I was at a fork in the road. I needed to choose to show up each day and do something, regardless of how small. Or I could choose to feel miserable. Giving up and showing up are just a breath apart. Sure, I was afraid of failing. I was replacing old habits with new ones and failures happen. If I learn from the failures, then they are as important as the successes."

Neo sighs, "I'm reading all your essays. That must count for something."

Dr. C. takes a seat. "Neo, I'm so glad you are finding them

useful. Awareness and learning new ways are the first steps toward a life with more moments of well-being. But to move forward, you need to show up ready to turn what you know into an action plan that is specifically tailored to your situation. It's a fork in the road offering the possibility to live better with a chronic illness."

"Yeah I know, wellness map. I got one from our healing relationship. But things have gotten worse and there's so many illness related problems. I just can't do it all." Neo's voice fades off into a soft whimper.

Reaching out to Neo in a gesture of support, Dr. C. says, "Feeling like you can't do it is much different than physically not being capable. From the darkness, or even partial darkness, it is hard to navigate. Especially if one is using the old coping habits."

"Think of it this way. You're traveling in a new car and you get a flat tire. The new car is the new face you have, and the flat tire represents those coping skills that used to wheel you along in life. The tire's gone flat because the old coping skills no longer work with the new face."

"Now you can choose to continue driving on the flat tire. Anyone who's tried this knows how difficult it is, even hazardous. You can choose to sit in your car on the side of the road and do nothing. Just give up. Or you can choose to take actions that get you moving again. Don't think of the entire trip. Just take the first step toward fixing the flat."

Mrs. Dr. C. sees Neo and Dr. C. in deep conversation. "Oh, Neo," she exclaims. "You look like you're struggling."

Neo glances up, "Dr. C. is helping me change my flat tire."

"That's great. I know for a fact that Dr. C. had a couple of flat tires over the last month. It started when, on a really bad day, he felt compelled to wield a pickaxe and enlarge the drainage ditch along the driveway." Mrs. Dr. C. sighs. "He knows this is dangerous for him. But those old habits of pushing through and doing too much were inescapable. He suffered greatly over the following week with muscle weakness, stiffness, and pain. It flattened all his tires."

Neo looks at Dr. C. and Dr. C. smiles sheepishly, "She's right, you know," says Dr. C. "I really knew better. But it just seemed so important at the time to get it done. I can be my worst enemy. Undue stress to the body from any source can create problems. I know I need to practice the whole rehab program described in my writing, but there are days when I fail."

Neo smiles and reaches out to Dr. C. "You and I will work together on wearing the new face. And we will 'show up' and not give up. Just let me know where you keep the tire jack for the next flat tire."

Loud Emotions Can Be Risky

They all stood and watched as the dog ran through my gardens trampling the newly transplanted iris and hosta. Neighbors called for their poorly trained dog to come. It did not. It kept up its role as canine tank. I love my gardens. I put a lot of sweat into creating a sanctuary that adds to my well-being. Standing by and watching it damaged was maddening. I think I have a right to be upset.

No matter how hard I work on living better with a chronic illness, something comes along to upset the apple cart. It's very frustrating to work so hard on improving and then something happens, some event outside of my control, to mess up the whole thing. I kept saying things like, "I really don't need this in my life." "This just isn't fair." "Why does it have to be my problem?" As the event consumed my thoughts, revisiting the event in my mind, I also connected it to past similar events.

Yes, the dog has trampled through the gardens before, and

failed to respond to its owner. I even wrote up a set of dog training instructions, with illustrations, and bought a dog whistle to attempt a solution. It didn't work. Now my brain was fluctuating back and forth between the collection of memories about the event and my search for a solution. I played out various scenarios in my brain while still being upset at the fact that I even had to come up with one. More emotions pushing me even closer to my threshold.

The closer I got to my threshold, the darker it became. I have written about the concept of darkness as a form of "brain blindness," triggered by emotions (especially those linked to self-survival). The sanctuary for me is part of my healthy survival with a chronic illness. The dog could become a threat to my survival.

Even though I knew I was approaching the dangerous threshold, I couldn't let it go. I felt justified in staying angry. This was an injustice. Something had to be done. My thrashing with the problem morphed into stomping around the house. I failed to communicate what I was going through to Mrs. Dr. C. The conversation started to get unnecessarily heated and I had to time myself out. It is what I call "spilling out behavior" – one of the first signs that the darkness is making itself known. I removed myself from the scene and didn't talk to Mrs. Dr. C. again until the morning.

Many times, we are often left to fix our own problems. These loud emotional situations are difficult for Mrs. Dr. C. I can't go to the neighbor and express my dismay with the level of intensity that I am feeling. If I am in a state of emotional upheaval, it falls to her to help defuse the situation, help me find a solution, and support and encourage me.

Research by the University of Sydney, Australia[176]

---

[176] Naismith, S.L., Pereira, M., Shine, J.M. and Lewis, S.J. "How well do caregivers detect mild cognitive change in Parkinson's disease?." *Movement Disorders*, 26 (2011): 161-164.

identified that in a group of 61 non-demented patients with Parkinson's disease, 62% met the criteria for mild cognitive impairment. The study also recognized that "the capacity for caregivers to rate mild cognitive change in PD may be useful to assist in early screening and intervention approaches." Partners of folks with PD can be of assistance. Those of us who have these mild cognitive processing problems can learn to recognize the brain blindness and accept the help. Mrs. Dr. C. and I have developed a communication strategy that helps us navigate these dark and stormy waters together.

This process of recycling a traumatic event, intensifying its emotive value, and connecting it to other similar events is what the brain does. Searching for patterns in all those events is what the brain does. Searching for a solution is what the brain does.

Our brains are not that great for accurate long-term memory storage (thank heavens for computers), but we are built for pattern recognition and solution generation. It is what our brain does naturally because it is designed that way. Although going back and forth between past and future is something natural to the brain, it becomes a problem when it doesn't function well. It's a problem when the whole process become unbalanced and out of control.

Loud emotions can be risky. The solution can be found in changing my reactions and training the brain to use the conductor to redirect the brain input. It's the new face of PD for me.

Brain Training Using the Conductor

Imagine that it is a bad day, and you are also in a PD "off period." Normally, it would be time to rest, right? But what if family arrives for dinner? It was the only time they could manage in their busy lives, and I really wanted to see them. The only solution was to find a way to manage the stimuli chaos flooding into my brain, being mindful of all motor movements, and presenting myself as social and civil. I was able to do it using the conductor. My only small cognitive error was mixing up people's names. Otherwise, it was a major accomplishment. Afterwards, I was exhausted for several days.

I am just beginning to understand how the conductor works to help with those awfully bad days. It takes time to learn how to apply the conductor in a way that replaces old habits like "fixing the flat tire." There are times when I say to myself, "You know this will pass. You know it doesn't stay this bad all the time. You know you will have good days. Your job right now, in the middle of the worst of it, is to tell those around you where you are and to practice holding the pause for the conductor."

The conductor idea has been mentioned in several essays as something I use to help me cope with Parkinson's disease. The conductor is an important part of that new face I have implemented. The conductor idea stems back to the idea of deep brain stimulation: Can the brain do its own modified form of DBS using a conductor (a mental construct) to moderate the signals coming into the brain?

We already have something like that in our brains – an ability to self-monitor while engaged in thinking/feeling/acting so we don't spill out our emotions. It is our ability to observe ourselves with genuine non-judgmental curiosity while also holding a pause between impulse and reaction.

In that pause is the doorway to a calm mind through meditation. The calm mind helps expand the pause, helps to strengthen it against intrusion. How we frame that pause shapes how it is used. If it is calmness that we seek, then it is that which will be discovered in the pause. This application of intent is part of the conductor's role. We can direct that intent at discovering ways of living better in the moment regardless of what else is there. My new face reflects the belief that there are always undiscovered possibilities within the expanded pause.

For the conductor to have a good chance of success, there must be a pause in the normal stream of consciousness which allows a shift to that perspective. There are many resources we draw from, giving us the energy needed to hold the pause and extend both its duration and its resistance to interference. Every moment of the day, we either add to this energy reserve or withdraw from it. It is about the little things every day. Every day, I am redirecting my actions, thoughts, and feelings away from that which makes me sicker. I am moving towards a healthier life. My full-time job now is learning how to live better with a chronic disease. I am not looking for a quick fix. I am looking to retrain my brain.

Here is an easy exercise. Get your body in a comfortable position and relax. This is not a contest and only works if you are completely relaxed. It is breathing in a way that engages the conductor and leads to a calm mind:

Counting Breath Exercise

When breathing in, you will say (at a mildly slow pace), "One thousand and one."

When breathing out (a little slower and deeper than normal), you will mentally count at a normal rate, "One...two...three..." and count until you finish the exhale. Don't push the breath. Be relaxed.

Next, continue the in breath with the next count, "One thousand and two" followed by counting on the out breath.

Repeat while counting.

If your thoughts or feelings intrude, causing you to stop counting, then observe why and start the in breath count again, "One thousand and one."

I have done this exercise during the worst of times and it was hard, but I was still able to keep track of progress. Remember, there is the relaxed pause (the conductor) and the intent of curious non-judgmental observations. Try it. How far can you count on the in breath before losing track and starting over? What caused you to lose track? How many counts happen on the out breath and what impacts that?

These are the beginning steps of conductor brain training and its application toward learning how to live better with PD. This counting breath exercise is deceptively simple. The next essay provides more detail. It takes months of practice to move beyond the first attempt to understanding the rich benefits of continued effort.

Conductor Training Helps Manage PD Symptoms

Conductor brain training has made living with PD easier for me. The most amazing thing I discovered using the conductor is that signals coming into my brain are sometimes distorted. This distortion can take place in the form of signal amplification or suppression. If I react to this distorted brain input as if it is real, then there are consequences that steal time away from the rehabilitation work. The second most amazing thing I discovered was that I can use my brain (specifically the conductor) to help manage symptoms.

Before I got Parkinson's, I was an upbeat positive guy with no signs of depression. Like so many others with PD, I have had to deal with input into my brain that feels like sadness. But when I use the conductor, I see from that view that there is nothing behind the sadness. There is no context. That's the disease speaking.

My brain wants to make context. That's what the brain

does. If the conductor were not in place, I'm almost sure it would do so. Instead, the conductor provides a fresh look at depression. This is a big deal for me. It is this shift in perspective, seeing the input as exaggerated, which has made a big impact.

The conductor helps us with the daunting tasks of learning how to do things all over again, even simple things like walking or eating. The conductor is useful in helping me cope with more PD symptoms than just depression. A well-trained conductor can help with the following:

- Appropriate exercise and fall prevention using mindful movements
- Managing chronic pain
- Decreasing impulsivity problems
- Improved mouth motor movement
- Get through the bad days and the off periods a bit easier

When I put the conductor in place to help with these symptoms, I find I am replacing old coping skills with new ones. I am fixing the "flat tire," retraining my brain, which results in a higher quality of life.

Learning how to use the conductor to help alleviate symptoms takes practice – lots of practice. In addition, it's important that this practice happens using a well-prepared brain. It is not easy to focus sustained attention on using the conductor while simultaneously engaging in life. I have found that exercise, little things practice, and the CHRONDI wellness mapmaking practices all contribute to preparing my brain for engaging the conductor.

The counting breath exercise is an easy way to be introduced to the conductor. It's important to follow the instructions as given. Of special importance is the intent held while doing the exercise. The conductor is non-judgmental, kind, and curious without causing harm.

It is also important to make mental note of the intrusions

which result in losing count of the in breath. Store this in memory and then go back to the counting breath exercise. You will retrieve this useful information later. There is also useful information in how many numbers are counted in the out breath. After you have done the counting breath exercise for a few weeks you may discover that the numbers counted in the out breath changes. Noting what affects these changes is important conductor brain training information.

There are times when this exercise and the conductor function poorly. These are when one crosses the emotion management threshold or enter the darkness, when deep fatigue sets in, when the brain is flooded with unhealthy chemicals (like alcohol or a poor medication choice), or if there is a brain injury. My wellness map includes instructions for me on how to avoid these dangers. Now I am practicing those instructions. Sometimes succeeding, sometimes failing, and always revising the wellness map accordingly.

This use of the conductor described here is a mental construct I use to help with PD symptom management. It is my way of describing self-care. It's a case study of one person and needs to be evaluated accordingly.

There are single case studies in the annals of brain science which made an impact, such as Phineas Gage who lived after having an iron bar blasted through the front part of his brain and "H.M." who had his hippocampus (a structure in the middle of the brain) snipped while fencing because his opponent's rapier sliced through his nose and into the brain. Science learned from these survivors of freak accidents. Anomalies become helpful to science only when we take the time to examine them.

Perfect Storm and Preventing Conductor Malfunction

It was one of those "perfect storm" weeks. You know, where everything comes together in a cumulative effect to make life miserable. When there is too much stress on my system, it is exceedingly difficult to use the conductor due to malfunctions. It only happens to me a few times a year. But it is quite disabling when it does.

The conductor is a mental construct where I can view my thoughts/feelings/actions in a relaxed state, and then direct my reactions to those thoughts, feelings, and actions. In the middle of the perfect storm being bombarded by pain, fatigue, over-the-top emotions, and the overwhelming urge to make it all go away, I really want to get up and escape. But movement causes great pain. The muscles are rigid, some in spasm. They are moving too slow, and don't always obey my commands. It takes almost all my energy simply to lie in bed and quiet my mind. Practice the counting breath exercise.

Most of the time, I can do the exercise. But not in the middle of the perfect storm. I tried. Got to the count of three. Then I watched as I said to myself, "Why am I doing this counting thing? There are more important things to pay attention to." Perfect storm weeks are filled with events that have strong emotional value. Like the story of the dog encounter, when I placed a sense of my own survival on an event.

I'm doing the same inside the perfect storm; I knew I was headed into dangerous waters. Most of the time, I can turn the rudder and redirect myself, so I don't end up spinning into the whirlpool of anxiety and depression. But not this time. I sailed over the threshold. It was a long night with the worst depression since losing my vision.

The conductor doesn't work well after crossing the

threshold of emotion management. It doesn't work well from inside the darkness. It doesn't work well if I have used my energy reserves and don't have enough to hold the pause for the conductor. It doesn't work well if the brain areas responsible for its function are damaged. These conductor malfunction situations are dangerous. I have developed a new attitude toward recuperative rest and not "doing." Yeah, that's right – Dr. C. doing "nothing" helps build the energy reserves back up so I can return to brain conductor training.

It takes a day or two to recover from navigating through the perfect storm. During those recovery days, it may appear to some that I am doing nothing. Sometimes I feel that way, like I am doing "nothing." I am not being productive in any usual sense of the term. I don't handle down time well, but I equate "doing" with accomplishing something tangible. That view has changed. For the first time since being a child, I understand the significance of recuperative down time. I need the time to heal myself. It is too risky walking around with a malfunctioning conductor and it just feels awful.

There is another risk – apparent apathy. Lie around sedentary for just a few days and this sensation of apathy kicks in. I call it apparent because there are sensations below the apathy – motor hesitancy, set shifting difficulty, thoughts that "I can't do it," and the uncomfortableness of moving muscles that have been still. All these sensations can become exaggerated because of PD. Using the conductor, I can strip away the illusion. Then, given that I am mostly recovered from the perfect storm, I find something motivating to get me active again. I can get stuck being sedentary and feeling apathetic, but my conductor sees it as just another reaction to distorted brain stimuli input.

If there is a perfect storm, then my job is to heal from its effects, stop being stuck, and get back to my wellness map – especially conductor brain training and appropriate exercise. It becomes a commitment, something that is in my life every day. It is also a sacred healing process and held that way when I am using it.

There are several essays in this book that address exaggerated emotion. I think it is a topic not clearly understood, and not well treated, in connection to Parkinson's disease.

A Fresh Look at Hallucinations and Parkinson's

A loud *crack*. I turned and yelled at my grandson, "Keep the billiard balls on the table." The noise was so loud that I was sure the ball had smashed into the sheetrock wall. I've been known to bounce a ball off the table practicing a special billiard shot. But the ball was still on the table. The noise was from a normal shot, with a touch of enthusiastic child play. Was this an auditory hallucination associated with PD?[177]

I have a tingling feeling on my feet that causes me to think there is an insect there. I swat my foot and check. Nothing there. I double check because I don't like spiders. Is that a tactile hallucination due to PD?[178]

Shadows out of the corner of my eye appear as a moving object, but on closer exam I discover nothing. Everyone does that. I'm not hallucinating, right?

Sensory hallucinations are known to be associated with

---

[177] Auditory: Inzelberg R., Kipervasser S., Korczyn A.D. "Auditory hallucinations in Parkinson's disease." *Journal of Neurology, Neurosurgery & Psychiatry* 1998; 64: 533-535.

[178] Tactile: Kataoka, Hiroshi, and Satoshi Ueno. "A review of tactile hallucinations in Parkinson's Disease." *Neuropsychiatry* Volume 7, Issue 3 (2017): 224-227.

PD[179] and can be early signs of psychosis.[180] Investigations on pre-levodopa administration suggest the link between PD and hallucinations existed before levodopa side effects.[181] Maybe this non-motor symptom of PD doesn't develop instantly as a psychosis but gradually worsens in that direction. In the early stages of PD, perhaps the hallucinations are very mild.

There is a difference between hallucinations, minor hallucinations, and pseudo hallucinations.[182] A hallucination is perceiving a sensation that does not correlate with reality and yet believing that it does – like the billiard ball incident. I believed that the ball came off the table and hit the wall. I saw it in my mind. If I swat at a bug that isn't there, then that seems to fit the definition. The shadow experience (a common phenomenon) is more of a pseudo hallucination because I really don't think there is something in the shadows, but I am going to check just to be sure.

I get feelings of depression which have no contextual foundation. The feeling can appear quite real, and if not managed, can become real. If there is no context (no real event in my life to cause me to feel depressed), then the internal

[179] General: Gilles Fénelon, Florence Mahieux, Renaud Huon, Marc Ziégler, "Hallucinations in Parkinson's disease: Prevalence, phenomenology and risk factors," *Brain*, Volume 123, Issue 4, April 2000, Pages 733-745, https://doi.org/10.1093/brain/123.4.733

[180] Psychosis: B R Thanvi, T C N Lo, D P Harsh. "Psychosis in Parkinson's Disease." *Postgrad Med J* 2005;81:644–646. doi: 10.1136/pgmj.2004.032029

[181] Pre levodopa: Gilles Fénelon, Christopher G. Goetz, Axel Karenberg. "Hallucinations in Parkinson disease in the prelevodopa era." *Neurology* Jan 2006, 66 (1) 93-98; DOI: 10.1212/01.wnl.0000191325.31068.c4

[182] Abhishek Lenka, Javier Pagonabarraga, Pramod Kumar Pal, Helena Bejr-Kasem, Jaime Kulisvesky. "Minor hallucinations in Parkinson disease: A subtle symptom with major clinical implications." *Neurology* Aug 2019, 93 (6) 259-266; DOI: 10.1212/WNL.0000000000007913

stimulus creating a feeling of depression is a hallucination of sorts. If I believe in the depressed feeling, then it's a hallucination. If not, then a pseudo hallucination.

Integrating a hallucination into my worldview can happen if I don't use the conductor. The conductor is a mental construct I use to observe cognitive processes and direct change. By using a strong conductor, I can strip away the illusion and see the depression input for what it truly is – faulty input. There are days when my conductor is malfunctioning. For a short period of time, I will be doing the "dance of darkness," oblivious to the dangers that come with believing in hallucinations.

I had a "first meet" exam with a new neurologist since moving to our new home. I always dread the first meeting because of the non-tremor, mostly hidden, nature of my Parkinson's disease. When asked if I hallucinate, I paused before answering. Exaggerated sensory input happens to me all the time. Now, I am training my conductor to evaluate before seeking context and reacting.

Because of the conductor, most of the exaggerated stimuli stay just that. Occasionally, some stimuli sneak through and get incorporated into the search for finding context to make sense of it all. I know about the signal distortion and its effect on how I direct my attention. It becomes a pseudo hallucination, not a hallucination. It's hard work to keep the conductor in place all the time, but it's a great benefit when I can use it.

I told the doctor I don't hallucinate, even though I experience exaggerated signal input several times a day. I probably should have said, "I have pseudo hallucinations." But that's a longer discussion about how PD and I live together. It's a discussion about how a well-trained conductor can change how we process adherent brain input. It's about pausing for the conductor immediately following exaggerated signal input.

I didn't know that when I reacted automatically to my grandson's enthusiastic billiard playing a few years past. I didn't know that my brain was lying to me. Most importantly, I didn't know that something could be done to strengthen the lie detector – the conductor.

Life History May Lead to a Strong Conductor

The conductor is a mental construct which supports metacognitive processes while in a rested state. That means it is a non-judgmental observer of the mind that is curious without causing harm. There are many benefits to having a strong conductor. But for me, the most beneficial is the "mind palace." I use the mind palace when writing these essays. The essays are often crafted without the first paragraph. I then go to the mind palace and, while holding the unfinished essay in working memory, I try out different beginnings and keep trying until I find ones I like. Wherever you take your mind throughout your life will shape what it becomes.

Another interesting use of the conductor is lucid dreaming – a form of metacognition. When neurologists ask me if I act out my dreams, I stumble with my answer. Yes, I have been known to move my arms or legs while in a dream. But I see myself doing it because of lucid dreaming. And then I stop. My answer has always been, "I've moved a bit while dreaming that I was stepping up." There is no research I could find that speaks to the role lucid dreaming and managing PD symptoms. I see it as evidence of a strong conductor, but it is one piece of many.

There is another skill that has a symbiotic relationship with the conductor skill. That is empathy. My Ph.D. research explored the idea that there could be an advanced form of empathy. I see empathy as a way of deeply connecting to others for the sole purpose of helping with suffering. Empathy is sitting with someone and letting go of interference so I can experience the connection with the other genuinely. With advanced empathy, it is as if I am really experiencing with the other (rather than role-playing my interpretation). This advanced empathy is part of the healing relationship, and it relies on a strong conductor to sit in an egoless place with the suffering of another.

The conductor also plays a role in creativity. Due to my life's paths, I became a theoretician. Basically, that is a person who comes up with a better way to explain things. Sometimes, this involves the synthesis of information into something new. But often it requires a leap, a fresh look. To step out of whatever conventional view I may have on the topic, I need to shift my perspective; reframe, change my mindset. Shifting mental perspectives is one of the main roles of the conductor. As a theoretician, it was something I often needed to do. It was cumbersome and awkward at first. Eventually, perspective shifting became a frequently used tool.

An important part of shifting perspective is the deep-seated intent we bring to the process. Therefore, I find holding a sacred intent as important and linked to a strong conductor. My "fresh look" essays each illustrate this shift in perspective. These shifts were also discovered while holding the intent of well-being for all. I seek to hold a sacred intent with everything I do – internally and externally. But, as I sometimes fail, I learn from that failure to not repeat it. There is no perfection. That is an illusion. I grow, fail, then develop and find some new tool to help me. There is an ethereal quality imparted to the process when a sacred intent is held in place by the conductor. Leaps of faith can happen.

Finally, I think that to be motivated in life toward building a strong conductor, there needs to be a reward or a sense of pleasure attached for using the conductor. The reward encourages practice, and the practice spurs skill development, which then triggers more reward. Sometimes, the reward is internally generated by bliss connected to creativity and well-being moments scattered along the journey. There are other times that the reward comes from the community because of the use of the conductor. It's in the smile of those you help. The reward by itself should never be pursued. Doing so puts in place a different intent and thus changes the outcome. The reward should always be a surprise. It takes lots of practice to develop a strong conductor with sacred intent held along the way. It is not self-serving. I am not looking to feel better. I'm looking to function better.

I am deeply grateful for all the opportunities that have woven together a life capable of presenting the important story of the brain's conductor and its possible role in helping people with PD.

My Parkinson's Portrait

During my Marine Corps training at Camp Lejeune, I was exposed to toxic chemicals in the water. It was not until the VA investigated[183] that Parkinson's was found to be strongly associated with this toxic chemical exposure. Out of the flames and into the fire, I was thrown into the jungles of Vietnam, where toxic chemicals were heavily used.[184] "The US program,

---

[183] *Committee on the Review of Clinical Guidance for the Care of Health Conditions Identified by the Camp Lejeune Legislation*; Board on the Health of Select Populations; Institute of Medicine. Review of VA Clinical Guidance for the Health Conditions Identified by the Camp Lejeune Legislation. Washington (DC): National Academies Press (US); 2015 Mar 26. 3, Characterization of Neurobehavioral Effects. Available from: https://www.ncbi.nlm.nih.gov/books/NBK284982/

[184] Parkinson's Foundation. Agent Orange & Other Toxic Exposures. Published on *Living With Parkinson's, Managing Parkinson's, Veterans and Parkinson's Disease*, undated.

codenamed 'Operation: Ranch Hand,' sprayed more than 20 million gallons of various herbicides over Vietnam, Cambodia, and Laos from 1961 to 1971."[185] The Da Nang and Quang Tri provinces, where I was deployed, were among the most heavily sprayed areas with Agent Orange.[186]

The connection between my symptoms and Parkinson's disease was not made easily. In the early stages of the disease, I was given a multitude of diagnoses and treatments. Most treatments did not work. Tests were inconclusive, although they showed abnormal results most of the time. Diagnoses of potassium deficiency, familial partial paralysis, MS, and "stick man disease" were thrown around like spaghetti on the wall hoping it will stick. Nothing fit and it was very discouraging.

The symptoms began interfering with work in 2004 and finally forced me to quit teaching (which I loved) in 2014. That same year, I was diagnosed with Parkinson's disease. The diagnosing physician did try the "gold standard" test of administering levodopa. The difference in my functioning was incredible. Since then, the progression in the disease has been slow, for which I am grateful.

I do not present with the classic PD symptoms identified over 200 years ago that neurologists identify as the "only" presentation of Parkinson's. It is interesting to note that James Parkinson reported "on six case sketches, three of the patients observed in the streets of London and one only seen from a distance."[187] Imagine that modern science in the 21st century

---

[185] A&E Television Networks. History.com. "Agent Orange," updated May 16, 2019.

[186] Twelve provinces were the most heavily sprayed with Agent Orange during the war. Ten of them cluster around one of the three air bases that became the most contaminate with dioxin: Da Nang, Phu Cat, and Bien Hoa. Published by Aspen Institute. Maps of Heavily Sprayed Areas and Dioxin Hot Spots.

[187] Goetz, Christopher G. "The history of Parkinson's disease: early clinical descriptions and neurological therapies." *Cold Spring Harbor*

continues to cling to a diagnosis proposed from observing only six cases in 1817. It's not the fault of the doctors. Our science has been lagging.

To date, there is not a better diagnostic match for the symptoms I present:

Persistent Symptoms

- Muscle pain and rigidity; dystonia in my legs at night or early morning
- Increased swallowing difficulty, aspiration of liquids
- Excessive sweating with poor homeostasis regulation
- An increasing intolerance to cold and heat
- Restlessness and sleep problems of insomnia and acting out motor movement
- Circadian rhythm disruption with episodes of prolonged wakefulness late in the night
- Hypersensitivity to sound
- Numbness and tingling beginning on the right side with right foot drag now also on the left side
- TMJ and nocturnal bruxism, with muscle spasms on the right side of my face
- Surges of sadness and anxiety with emotional lability which have no context and occur daily during the off periods
- Reduction in eye blinking

Episodic Symptoms

- Episodes of slowed movement along with decrease in motor coordination due to amplitude control issues – the constant missing to grasp objects with intentional effort or dropping things unintentionally
- Episodic constipation and abdominal cramping, urinary retention
- Episodic drooling with orgasm; erectile dysfunction

perspectives in medicine vol. 1,1 (2011): a008862. doi:10.1101/cshperspect.a008862

- Episodes of deep fatigue accompanied by a decrease in cognitive performance

Neurologists have documented the "cog wheel effect" on the right arm. I teeter with an unstable walking when doing toe to heel pattern, but normal in other balance and walking tests conducted in the office. At home, however, balance seems to elude me on some occasions. Getting up out of bed produces wobbles, as does rising from my office chair or the couch.

Then there is other clinical evidence reported by other specialties that link their expert diagnostic skills with manifestations known in Parkinson's (urology, ophthalmology).

I shared an incident with my new neurologist which happened just after we finished relocating. I had non-exertional shortness of breath. I wanted to be sure it wasn't COVID. But something unusual happened at the ER. I was chatting with the doc and then he said to me, "You can put your arms down now." I looked and saw that indeed my arms were frozen in midair.

I had a DaTscan looking for PD-related brain damage two years ago. My results were negative. But then, a major portion of brain must be affected to be positive. The common assumption is that progression must happen at a pace which shows dramatic worsening in PD patients five years after initial diagnosis. That hasn't happened with me. My progression seems to be starting now, 10 years after diagnosis. It accelerates in fits and starts but ultimately, once a symptom develops, it stays with me.

Much of my writing is about early detection and treatment of PD. If providers are looking for the patient to fit into this feeble old guy PD stereotype, then how is it ever going to be possible to do early detection and treatment? When a physician rejects the symptoms or the findings of other specialists, I ask, "Well, what do you think is going on?" I am most often answered by silence. It's not the doctor's fault. The science is missing something.

For patients like me who have non-tremor PD, we need the door held open to the possibility of a form of PD which falls outside the classic criteria – particularly if we seek early detection and adequate treatment.

The Insular Cortex Dopamine Center and its Relationship to PD

My idea of *Possibilities with Parkinson's* began with just trying to understand what is happening to me. Since I do not display the dramatic motor symptoms of Parkinson's disease (but have many of the non-motor symptoms), I seek out research that can help explain what I am experiencing. Medical providers who don't see the classic symptoms really shut down conversations about what is going on in my brain and in my body. For me, it is time to take control.

While researching dopamine neurons, I found the new MRI technique out of MIT that showed whole brain dopamine utilization.[188] When the whole brain is scanned looking at dopamine use, it becomes clear that there are not one, but two major dopamine areas in the brain.

First is the region that gives us the classic symptoms involving the motor cortex and connecting midbrain

---

[188] "How dopamine drives brain activity. A specialized MRI sensor reveals the neurotransmitter's influence on neural activity throughout the brain." Anne Trafton, *MIT News Office*. Published April 1, 2020.
See also: "How dopamine drives brain activity." McGovern Institute, April 1, 2020. First published as Li, N., Jasanoff, A. "Local and global consequences of reward-evoked striatal dopamine release." *Nature* 580, 239-244 (2020).

structures.[189] The second is the insular cortex. When not functioning properly, the insular cortex can result in many of the non-motor symptoms associated with PD, including many that I experience.

The researchers at MIT are not the first to link the insular cortex to dopamine and PD symptoms. A 2014 summary of the connection to non-motor PD symptoms[190] states that the insular cortex is:

"Highly involved in integrating somatosensory, autonomic, and cognitive-affective information to guide behavior. Thus, it acts as a central hub for processing relevant information related to the state of the body as well as cognitive and mood states. Despite these crucial functions, the insula has been largely overlooked as a potential key region in contributing to non-motor symptoms of Parkinson's disease. The insula is affected in Parkinson's disease by alpha-synuclein deposition, disruptions in normal neurotransmitter function, alterations in connectivity as well as metabolic and structural changes. Although research focusing on the role in Parkinson's disease is scarce, there is evidence from neuroimaging studies linking the insula to cognitive decline, behavioral abnormalities, and somatosensory disturbances."

A more recent paper[191] provides another overview of the roles served by the insular cortex:

---

[189] Burciu, Roxana G. PhD, Vaillancourt, David E. PhD. "Imaging of Motor Cortex Physiology in Parkinson's Disease." *Movement Disorders*, Volume 33, Issue 11, 1688-1699. November 2018.
[190] Christopher, Leigh, et al. "Uncovering the role of the insula in non-motor symptoms of Parkinson's disease." *Brain*, Volume 137, Issue 8, August 2014, Pages 2143–2154, https://doi.org/10.1093/brain/awu084
[191] Benarroch, Eduardo E. "Insular cortex: Functional complexity and clinical correlations." *Neurology*, November 2019, 93 (21) 932-938; DOI: 10.1212/WNL.0000000000008525

"The posterior (granular) insula receives inputs from pain, temperature, visceral, vestibular, and other sensory pathways; this multimodal sensory representation is further elaborated in the midinsular (dysgranular) cortex and then conveyed to the anterior (agranular) insula, which further processes this information and interacts with areas involved in cognitive and emotional control. The insula thus provides an interface between bodily sensation and emotion and may have a key role in perceptual awareness, social behavior, and decision making."

In other words, the insular cortex is involved in states of consciousness, in particular switching between thinking, planning, and emotions.[192] It plays a role in autopilot function, internal body perception – such as pain[193] and homeostasis – and emotion management in goal-directed behavior.[194] It serves as a buffer between incoming sensory input and higher cortical functions aimed at goal attainment. Researchers hypothesize that impairment in insular cortex functioning is correlated with a progression in Parkinson's disease.[195]

---

[192] Li, Ruie, et al. "The fronto-insular cortex causally mediates the default-mode and central-executive networks to contribute to individual cognitive performance in healthy elderly." *Human Brain Mapping.* 2018; 39: 4302-4311. https://doi.org/10.1002/hbm.24247

[193] Martikainen IK, Hagelberg N, Jääskeläinen SK, Hietala J, Pertovaara A. "Dopaminergic and serotonergic mechanisms in the modulation of pain: In vivo studies in human brain." *Eur J Pharmacol.* 2018 Sep 5;834:337-345. doi: 10.1016/j.ejphar.2018.07.038. Epub 2018 Jul 20. PMID: 30036531.

[194] "Insular Cortex: Structure, Function & Role in Motivation." Study.com, published January 23, 2018, study.com/academy/ lesson/insular-cortex-structure-function-role-in-motivation.html

[195] Kikuchi, Akio, et al. "Hypoperfusion in the supplementary motor area, dorsolateral prefrontal cortex and insular cortex in Parkinson's disease." *Journal of the Neurological Sciences*, Volume 193, Issue 1, 2001, Pages 29-36, ISSN 0022-510X, https://doi.org/10.1016/S0022-510X(01)00641-4.

Clinical presentation of patients who have damage to the insular cortex can include the following:

- Difficulty moderating emotions, including anxiety and depression
- Hypersensitivity to sound[196]
- Breakdowns in autopilot functioning
- Problems maintaining homeostasis, like temperature regulation and sweating
- Circadian rhythm problems[197]
- Chronic pain

These are all symptoms present in my clinical portrait.[198] The science supports the idea that there is a second dopamine production area involved with Parkinson's disease – the insular cortex. If you are looking for more information, Nadine Gogolla did a nice overview of the insular cortex, its biology, and functions.[199]

What does this mean to me or you or any patient who experiences these symptoms, but does not demonstrate profound tremors or shaking? To be fair, the science of

---

[196] Boucher, Olivier, et al. "Hyperacusis following unilateral damage to the insular cortex: A three-case report."
Brain Research, Volume 1606, 2015, Pages 102-112, ISSN 0006-8993, https://doi.org/10.1016/ j.brainres. 2015.02.030.

[197] "Disrupted Circadian Rhythms Linked to Later Parkinson's Diagnosis. Researchers Probe Brain's 24-Hour Biological Clock for Neurodegenerative Risks." By Jeff Norris, published on UCSF Research, The University of California, San Francisco, June 15, 2020. Study first published: Leng Y, et al. "Association of Circadian Abnormalities in Older Adults with an Increased Risk of Developing Parkinson Disease." *JAMA Neurol.* 2020 Jun 15:e201623. doi: 10.1001/ jamaneurol.2020.1623. Epub ahead of print. PMID: 32539075; PMCID: PMC7296450.

[198] "My Parkinson's Portrait Is Outside the Classic Criteria." Dr. C. "Possibilities with Parkinson's" published on Parkinson's News Today, October 2, 2020.

[199] Gogolla, Nadine. "The insular cortex." *Current Biology*, Volume 27, Issue 12, 2017, Pages R580-R586, ISSN 0960-9822, https://doi.org/10.1016/j.cub.2017.05.010.

Parkinson's disease is not exact. It is being researched and studied, and for every posited determination of cause, more questions arise. There is so much we don't know.

I am a strong advocate of science. I was trained in two different domains to ask questions – and investigate occurrences, causes, and effects – in a systematic manner. As patients, we seek professional opinions to understand our diseases and seek treatment for symptoms. Ultimately, we are responsible for our own health. As we cannot assume innocence of knowing what impacts our health adversely, we must be responsible for what we can do better.

The Default Mode Network: Lies from the Insular Cortex

I have written about "the conductor,"[200] a mental construct useful for shifting perspective. The conductor likely has major neural components in a network of areas in the brain: the default mode network, the salience network, and the executive network. In this essay, I will focus on the default mode network and its link to the insular cortex. I believe possibilities for improving outcomes for patients with PD lie here.

Damage to the default mode network has been noted for PD patients.[201] The default mode network is connected to the insular cortex. The insular cortex acts as a switching gate between the default mode network, the salience network, and

[200] "Brain Training Using the Conductor." Dr. C. "Possibilities with Parkinson's," published on Parkinson's News Today, August 28, 2020
[201] van Eimeren, Thilo et al. "Dysfunction of the default mode network in Parkinson disease: a functional magnetic resonance imaging study." *Archives of neurology* vol. 66,7 (2009): 877-83. doi:10.1001/archneurol.2009.97

the executive network.[202] Switching performed by the insular cortex allows sensory input to be evaluated by the desired network. The analogy would be a train that the engineers direct down specific tracks to get to the right station – or avoid hitting other trains! "Hitting a train" equates, to us, a feeling of being overwhelmed. PD causes damage to the insular cortex.[203] I propose here that damage to the insular cortex, particularly the anterior portion, causes faulty sensory input.[204] Continually using this faulty input will, over time, result in new (but inaccurate) patterns of thoughts, feelings, and actions. These are the lies our brain tells us, which jeopardize our already difficult PD life.

Continual faulty processing in the brain can result in the PD person acting differently. I first experienced this in 2014. I overreacted to a student in class, not being able to control my emotional input in that social situation. It was the first time I did this in over 20 years of teaching. I wanted an answer as to why my brain was acting in a way so contrary to my history.

There is much clinical research about the default mode network. It is difficult to make sense of all the scientific and medical descriptions. Simply put, I label it "our resting mind state." I think of it as the place where our mind wanders during creativity and brainstorming, or the pause before using the conductor to observe thinking and enter deeper meditation. It is a place where one is mentally quiet so that the

---

[202] Putcha, Deepti et al. "Salience and Default Mode Network Coupling Predicts Cognition in Aging and Parkinson's Disease." *Journal of the International Neuropsychological Society : JINS* vol. 22,2 (2016): 205-15. doi:10.1017/ S1355617715000892

[203] "The Insular Cortex Dopamine Center and Its Relationship to Parkinson's." Dr. C. "Possibilities with Parkinson's, published on Parkinson's News Today, October 9, 2020.

[204] Wang, Xingchao et al. "Anterior insular cortex plays a critical role in interoceptive attention." *eLife,* vol. 8 e42265. 15 Apr. 2019, doi:10.7554/eLife.42265

mind can function without being constantly interrupted by a stream of sensory input.

I find it difficult to enter that resting mind state when my brain is being bombarded with exaggerated input. I experience this faulty input as surges of exaggerated emotion[205] and other symptoms.[206] We know that damage to the insular cortex affects functioning of the default mode network. It may also explain my recurring moments of depression or anxiety that I did not have prior to PD.

The insular cortex is considered a dopamine producing center. Why does the brain need it? PD patients lose dopamine constantly. I think my frequent use of the conductor helps access sources of this chemical so I can function better with PD.[207]

Being able to be a calm presence in social situations was always my strength. That ended with PD. Now, I must practice calmness, with exercise, and do so throughout the day. The further the disease progresses, the harder I need to work and show up every day ready to find the possibility in that day.

Calming down requires daily practice[208] in combination with exercise. I discovered a cleansing effect that combines the two. I can quiet down the insular cortex input. I can find the quiet resting mind. I have failed many times, but more importantly, I have also found that I can succeed.

---

[205] "Loud Emotions Can Be Risky. Here's How to Change Course." Dr. C. "Possibilities with Parkinson's," Published on Parkinson's News Today, August 21, 2020.

[206] "My Parkinson's Portrait Is Outside the Classic Criteria." Dr. C. "Possibilities with Parkinson's," Published on Parkinson's News Today, October 2, 2020.

[207] "Life's History Can Lead to a Strong Conductor." Dr. C. "Possibilities with Parkinson's," Published on Parkinson's News Today, September 25, 2020.

[208] "Brain Training Using the Conductor." Dr. C. "Possibilities with Parkinson's," Published on Parkinson's News Today, August 28, 2020.

As I practice quieting down that noisy input, I discovered I need to also relax my muscles. I practice a routine of stretching and massage before and after exercise and sometimes during bad off periods. When I combine this conductor/exercise training with a purposeful life guided by a sacred wellness map,[209] I find something new emerges. I'm not just calmer; I function better.

I believe that one of the functions of the default mode network (the conductor) is to instruct the insular cortex to dampen down the input. It buffers the sensory input. It is easier to be more productive and in control of my thinking and emotions when I use the conductor to quiet my mind. In activating this buffer, I believe I am also activating the dopamine producing neurons. I am not just calmer. Conductor/exercise practice decreases symptoms of PD that affect quality of life.

Conductor/exercise practice may also contribute to the slow disease progression I experience. I find comfort in understanding what PD is doing to me and what I can do to affect the negative outcomes. I believe it is an understanding that supports the running header on my columns – "Possibilities with Parkinson's."

Parkinson's Disease Remission: Can the Conductor Help?

Previous essays have discussed[210] using the conductor (in

[209] "The CHRONDI Creed: A Guide for Parkinson's Warriors." Dr. C. "Possibilities with Parkinson's," Published on Parkinson's News Today, February 8, 2019.

[210] "The Default Mode Network: Lies From the Insular Cortex." Dr. C. "Possibilities with Parkinson's," Published on Parkinson's News Today, October 16, 2020.

particular, the resting mind state) to suppress faulty input from the second dopamine center[211] and thus reduce the effects of PD symptoms. Is there any evidence to support this besides that which I find in my quest to understand?

The first piece of evidence is my own life with PD. We know there are dangers in applying medical scientific information to self-awareness. I would not recommend self-application without a strong conductor. Even then, one should be willing to have peer review. I present myself as a case of atypical non-tremor PD,[212] while at the same time having this unique life history that stimulated my brain to utilize the conductor.[213] Since the second dopamine center is broken, it occasionally sends me misinformation. A strong conductor helps me shift perspective and see the illusion being presented.

The conductor/exercise training provided throughout my life has enabled me to shift perspective, to look at things differently. It has been a part of seeking creative solutions and healing. That ability to shift perspective, combined with the training, has led me to share my story of possibilities with PD.

I am not the only case to show improvement with PD (or at least a slower than normal decline).[214]

---

[211] "The Insular Cortex Dopamine Center and Its Relationship to Parkinson's." Dr. C. "Possibilities with Parkinson's," Published on Parkinson's News Today, October 9, 2020.

[212] "My Parkinson's Portrait Is Outside the Classic Criteria." Dr. C. "Possibilities with Parkinson's," Published on Parkinson's News Today, October 2, 2020.

[213] "Life's History Can Lead to a Strong Conductor." Dr. C. "Possibilities with Parkinson's," Published on Parkinson's News Today, September 25, 2020.

[214] X, Wang L, Liu S, Zhu L, Loprinzi PD, Fan X. "The Impact of Mind-body Exercises on Motor Function, Depressive Symptoms, and Quality of Life in Parkinson's Disease: A Systematic Review and Meta-analysis." *Int J Environ Res Public Health.* 2019 Dec 18;17(1):31. doi: 10.3390/ijerph17010031. PMID: 31861456; PMCID: PMC6981975.

Medical literature reports a man who had PD and then he didn't.[215] Is this an example of PD remission? The authors offer as their explanation for why this change happened the fact that the man practiced meditation. I see meditation as involving a shift in perception through the resting mind state[216] and a role of the conductor.[217]

In her book *Radical Remission*,[218] Dr. Kelly Turner describes themes common throughout interviews with people who experienced radical remissions from cancer. Of the nine themes she identified, seven involved a shift in perception, e.g., taking charge of your health and discovering a deeper meaning or purpose. The brain can influence the body, as in the relaxation response used for addressing stress[219] and the use of mindfulness.[220] It may be that shifting perspective can be of benefit to people who have PD.

Shifts in perspective may be something that, when done with the proper intent over time, aid in the healing process. My research on advanced empathy describes a catharsis and a shift in perspective as part of what transpires within the healing relationship. The role of the conductor is to help with

[215] Smart, K., Durso, R., Morgan, J., McNamara, P. "A potential case of remission of Parkinson's disease." *J Complement Integr Med*. 2016 Sep 1;13(3):311-315. doi: 10.1515/jcim-2016-0019. PMID: 27379905.

[216] "The Default Mode Network: Lies From the Insular Cortex." Dr. C. "Possibilities with Parkinson's," Published on Parkinson's News Today, October 16, 2020.

[217] "Brain Training Using the Conductor." Dr. C. "Possibilities with Parkinson's," Published on Parkinson's News Today, August 28, 2020.

[218] Turner, Kelly A. *Radical Remission: Surviving Cancer Against All Odds*. HarperOne, 2014.

[219] Lazar S.W., Bush G., Gollub R.L., Fricchione G.L., Khalsa G., Benson H. "Functional brain mapping of the relaxation response and meditation." *Neuroreport*. 2000 May 15;11(7):1581-5. PMID: 10841380.

[220] Kabat-Zinn, Jon. *Full Catastrophe Living (Revised Edition): Using the Wisdom of Your Body and Mind to Face Stress, Pain, and Illness*. Bantum, September 24, 2013

shifts in perspective. My previous "A Fresh Look" essays offer several examples of using a shift in perspective to help with PD.

Conductor/exercise training doesn't have to be something special. It can be molded around almost any activity in daily life. One of the easiest ways to practice is being creative in something you like to do. Creativity here is defined as producing something that did not exist before, rather than reproducing what you created earlier. It may be that engaging in creative and new/novel tasks daily will strengthen the conductor because such mental efforts require a shift in perspective.

I have found that there is a symbiotic relationship between exercise and conductor training when it comes to managing my PD symptoms. Symbiotic training is more than one approach alone. It provides the healthy muscles needed to benefit from the conductor training. The body strengthens and the conductor strengthens. Exercise helps the brain get ready to heal. The two working in harmony provide more energy in the well of resources I draw from to get through each day. There are fewer severe off periods. Together, exercise and conductor training provide input into improved functioning and provide a reward feedback loop. That is the symbiotic relationship.

What I present here is not proof that conductor and exercise training always works to help people who have PD. A single case study, even with scientific support, cannot translate easily to a large population. This is an idea, a story of one man's life with PD and how he has made sense of things. I share what I do to offset the worst of what PD throws at me. Only the future will tell if my story has utility. What I do offer is possibility, and that can be the foot in the door helping to keep hope alive.

It's Time to Redefine Early-Stage PD

The symbiotic conductor/exercise training helps me live better with PD. Putting it in place as an early intervention (unknowingly on my part) was a crucial piece of this successful outcome. If we are to explore the utility of conductor/exercise training for others with PD, then we need to know what early PD looks like.

There is quite a buzz in the scientific literature about prodromal ("early") features of PD. Alexander Kilzheimer, lead author of "The Challenge and Opportunity to Diagnose Parkinson's Disease in Midlife", states:

"Its [Parkinson's disease] current clinical diagnosis is based on motor symptoms that appear late during disease progression when substantial proportions of the nigrostriatal dopaminergic neuron population are lost already. Although disturbances in sleep and other biofunctions often surface years prior to motor impairments and point to a long prodromal phase, these phenotypic signs in a person's midlife lack predictive power. They do, however, signal the unfolding of the disease and suggest molecular correlates that begin deviating early on. Revealing such trajectories, hence, promises not only a better understanding of prodromal PD but may also enable a much-needed earlier diagnosis."[221]

The disease is currently clinically defined by a set of cardinal motor features centered on the presence of bradykinesia and at least one additional motor symptom out of tremor, rigidity, or postural instability.

However, converging evidence from clinical, neuro-pathological, and imaging research suggests there may be

---

[221] Kilzheimer, Alexander, et al. "The Challenge and Opportunity to Diagnose Parkinson's Disease in Midlife." *Frontiers in neurology* vol. 10 1328. 17 Dec. 2019, doi:10.3389/fneur.2019.01328

initiation of PD-specific pathology prior to appearance of these classical motor signs. This latent phase of neurodegeneration in PD is of relevance in relation to the development of disease-modifying or neuroprotective therapies which would require intervention at the earliest stages of disease.

A key challenge in PD research, therefore, is to identify and validate markers for the preclinical and prodromal stages of the illness. Philipp Mahlknecht and his co-authors identify that many of these prodromal symptoms may precede the classic PD motor symptoms by as many as 10 to 20 years in some cases.[222]

Here is a brief list of possible new early-stage criteria:

Non-Motor Symptoms
- Reduced ability to smell
- Constipation

- Depression/anxiety
- Idiopathic REM sleep behavior
- Reduced executive function in brain

Motor Symptoms
- Reduced arm swing
- Changes in walking patterns (foot drag)
- Stiffness
- Tremor

- Slowed movements (bradykinesia)

I identified foot drag in a previous column as one of my early symptoms.[223] I have a rigid variation of Parkinson's and only a mild tremor. A study in early, nonmedicated PD patients by Ania Winogrodzka, et. al., states, "When the confounding influence of rigidity is taken into account, no significant direct relationship between dopaminergic

[222] Mahlknecht, Philipp, et al. "The Concept of Prodromal Parkinson's Disease." *Journal of Parkinson's disease,* vol. 5,4 (2015): 681-97. doi:10.3233/JPD-150685

[223] "Foot Problems as an Early Sign of PD: Oh, What a Drag It Is!" Dr. C. "Possibilities with Parkinson's," Published on Parkinson's News Today, December 7, 2018.

degeneration and the degree of tremor could be found."[224] If you're looking for a tremor, I don't demonstrate it consistently.

In addition to these symptoms, the new early stage might demonstrate episodic motor movement problems. Who hasn't done the finger-to-nose or repetitive finger-tapping test in the neurology office? Jennifer C. Uzochukwu and Elizabeth L. Stegemöller identify that:

"Changes in movement amplitude and movement rate may influence fine-motor dexterity tasks differently. Thus, it is important to consider the quantitative assessment of both movement rate and movement amplitude because they may indicate differential clinical applications in the treatment of people with PD."[225]

Ask me to repeat finger-to-nose, and I will only miss occasionally. I more often knock over the water cup, or bump into Mrs. Dr. C. while navigating through a narrow open space, because of a problem with movement amplitude regulation.[226] In other words, I'm prone to missing exactly where I intended to direct my arm, leg, or body. I can overreach, underreach, or just wobble enough to create havoc.

Pain has also been identified in the early stage and has

[224] Winogrodzka, Ania, et al. "Rigidity decreases resting tremor intensity in Parkinson's disease: A [(123)I]beta-CIT SPECT study in early, nonmedicated patients." *Movement Disorders.* 2001 Nov;16(6):1033-40. doi: 10.1002/mds.1205. PMID: 11748734.

[225] Uzochukwu, Jennifer C., and Elizabeth L. Stegemöller. "Repetitive Finger Movement and Dexterity Tasks in People with Parkinson's Disease." *American Journal of Occupational Therapy*, 04 2019, Vol. 73, 7303205090. https://doi.org/10.5014/ajot.2019.028738

[226] Mazzoni, Pietro, et al. "Motor control abnormalities in Parkinson's disease." *Cold Spring Harbor perspectives in medicine* vol. 2,6 (2012): a009282. doi:10.1101/cshperspect.a009282

been a topic of my columns.[227] Reported in Parkinson's News Today in 2018,[228] researchers at the Bangur Institute of Neurosciences in India conducted a combined hospital and community-based study and identified several PD-specific areas and nocturnal leg cramps. "This is an indirect evidence that pain can be an important early clinical marker of [Parkinson's]," the authors wrote.

Scientists are developing a better understanding PD and a new picture of early-stage PD is emerging, but it is still a fledgling science and there is a good chance my description of early-stage PD will have changes over time. The description of a new early stage is not the final description. As we expand our understanding of PD, the science will redefine the disease. The medical community predicts that improved research and recognition of prodromal symptoms will dramatically change the face of Parkinson's: "By 2040, it is hoped that prodromal criteria will be incorporated into active neuroprotective treatment programs, allowing a program of population-based screening followed by early treatment and ultimately the prevention of clinical PD from ever becoming manifest."[229]

---

[227] "Rewiring the Brain: Taking a Fresh Look at Chronic Pain." Dr. C. "Possibilities with Parkinson's," Published on Parkinson's News Today, July 10, 2020.

[228] "Pain May Be Early Detector of Parkinson's, Study Suggests." Jose Marques Lopes, PhD, in *News, Published on* Parkinson's News Today, August 27, 2018.

[229] Berg, Daniela, and Ronald B Postuma. "From Prodromal to Overt Parkinson's Disease: Towards a New Definition in the Year 2040." *Journal of Parkinson's disease* vol. 8,s1 (2018): S19-S23. doi:10.3233/JPD-181457

Conversations with Neo: One Brick at a Time

The imaginary conversational neocortex of my brain, whom I call Neo, looks up from reading my column, "Possibilities with Parkinson's."

"Hey, Doc. I still don't understand this conductor theory.[230] How can I use it as a treatment for our Parkinson's?" he asks, referring to a mental construct Dr. C. has developed to shift his perspective while managing Parkinson's.

"Hold on a minute, my friend." Dr. C. responds. "The conductor/exercise training[231] I've frequently written about is not a treatment yet. It's just one man's idea about an intervention that might help. More research needs to be done. I wouldn't even know how to scale it up to the larger population based only on my own experience."

"I think it's a cool idea, you know," Neo says. "Training our own brain to make dopamine."

Dr. C. settles into his chair.

"I may seem to suggest that, but what I really think is that we can slow the progression of Parkinson's and the severity of its symptoms by using conductor/exercise training," Dr. C. says. "If such a thing is possible, then it will be up to the medical research scientists to provide explanations.

"One of my important goals is to leave this world better than it was when I arrived," Dr. C adds. "Achieving this requires a long-term functioning conductor, and it plays an important role in goal-driven behavior.

"Any conductor/exercise training would need to be

---

230 "Brain Training Using the Conductor." Dr. C. "Possibilities with Parkinson's," Published on Parkinson's News Today, August 28, 2020.
231 "Conductor Training Can Help You Manage Parkinson's Symptoms." Dr. C. "Possibilities with Parkinson's," Published on Parkinson's News Today, September 4, 2020.

individually tailored to be of most benefit to an individual to meet their goals. Offering myself as a case study is risky on many levels, but it's just one piece of the whole picture. Information about a second dopamine center[232] is seeing new research, along with its impact on nonmotor Parkinson's symptoms[233] – many of which match my own.

"The scientific literature suggests that this second dopamine area is connected to the default mode network,[234] our resting mind state. This means we have a built-in mechanism for moderating the input coming from the second dopamine center. This is exemplified in my "Fresh Look"[235] columns about Parkinson's and pain, and Parkinson's-related depression.[236] My question is: If we engage this buffering mechanism, does it activate the dopamine neurons? I believe it does. And I believe the result is an improvement, or slower decrease, of some of the physical symptoms, as in my case.

"If you then add physical exercise,[237] the positive effects of both the conductor and exercise are enhanced.

"But I want to repeat: This is not a treatment. I am offering

[232] "The Insular Cortex Dopamine Center and Its Relationship to Parkinson's." Dr. C. "Possibilities with Parkinson's," Published on Parkinson's News Today, October 9, 2020.

[233] "My Parkinson's Portrait Is Outside the Classic Criteria." Dr. C. "Possibilities with Parkinson's," Published on Parkinson's News Today, October 2, 2020.

[234] "The Default Mode Network: Lies From the Insular Cortex." Dr. C. "Possibilities with Parkinson's," Published on Parkinson's News Today, October 16, 2020.

[235] "Rewiring the Brain: Taking a Fresh Look at Chronic Pain." Dr. C. "Possibilities with Parkinson's," Published on Parkinson's News Today, July 10, 2020.

[236] "A Fresh Look at Depression and Chronic Illness." Dr. C. "Possibilities with Parkinson's," Published on Parkinson's News Today, July 31, 2020.

[237] "Rethinking Exercise with Parkinson's." Dr. C. "Possibilities with Parkinson's," Published on Parkinson's News Today, June 26, 2020.

it as a case study of someone who might be an example of Parkinson's damage in the second dopamine center more than the more widely understood nigrostriatal area."

Neo looks a little confused. "OK. So, if it isn't a treatment, then what should we do with all of this information?"

"The early steps in using the conductor focus on developing and maintaining a pause between emotional or exaggerated sensory input, a pause before thought or action," Dr. C. replies.

"The pause allows the conductor to be utilized.[238] The idea is based on neural plasticity: If I stimulate the right pathways, then I can build a bridge around the damaged brain areas. The bridge I build in my brain won't look the same as the one someone else would build. It takes years of hard work to rewire the brain.

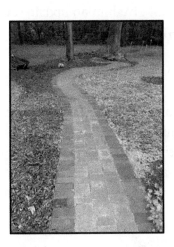

One brick at a time. (Photo by Darcy Hoisington)

"We have this saying at our house: 'one brick at a time.'

---

[238] "Conductor Training Can Help You Manage Parkinson's Symptoms." Dr. C. "Possibilities with Parkinson's," Published on Parkinson's News Today, September 4, 2020.

Keep at it every day, even if it's just one small thing a day, just one brick a day, and eventually it will turn into a path."

Mrs. Dr. C. chimes in: "I think I can give some testimony to Dr. C.'s efforts in training the conductor. I see fewer uncontrolled outbursts, and I see him taking stock of his emotions before he says or does something he might regret."

Neo laughs. "Dr. C. has outbursts? I can't picture that!"

"Oh yes," Mrs. Dr. C. says, smiling. "It used to be that the slightest provocation would trigger them. Now, we anticipate that he might have difficulty using the conductor in highly stressful situations. In general, day-to-day responses are managed. But it took him several years to do that."

"Of course," she adds wistfully, "we try to anticipate when a highly stressful situation might rear its ugly head. We try to space out appointments and commitments with enough time in between to rest. I give him an update several times during the week about what is coming up on the calendar. I guess you might say that I am helping his brain conductor know when the 'trains' are coming down the track."

"Perhaps I need a Mrs. Dr. C. to help me work on my brain conductor training," Neo says. "Maybe other Parkinson's caregivers or family members understand what this means so they can help their Parkinson's partner."

Dr. C. smiles at Mrs. Dr. C. "I can't imagine what I would do without her helping me lay one brick at a time."

Atypical Non-Tremor Parkinson's can be confused with PTSD

"You're a vet. All Vietnam vets have PTSD." Simple statements which somehow miss the mark in my case. Prior to being diagnosed with PD, I was not diagnosed with any of the symptoms attributable to PTSD. Despite having the PTSD ruled out by psychologists twice as part of the routine VA evaluation for disability, it still rears its ugly head. Yes, many vets have PTSD. However, I think there are just as many PD patients who have acquired similar symptoms like my case who have atypical non-tremor Parkinson's and not PTSD.

Previously, I suggested how PD might be causing PTSD[239] (largely due to the losses and stress involved[240]). With the discovery of a possible atypical non-tremor Parkinson's associated with a malfunctioning second dopamine center,[241] I have a fresh look on what might be happening to me.

I did not have life-altering anxiety prior to the PD diagnosis. For 40 years, I was a fully functioning member of society with decades of successful employment in several highly cognitive professions. It is the atypical non-tremor Parkinson's which causes symptoms that present like PTSD and add confusion in the diagnosis.

This next information is very clinical but worth reading. Here are the diagnostic criteria for PTSD:

The diagnostic criteria for DSM-5 PTSD include symptoms and signs grouped into five main clusters, including exposure to severe stress (Cluster A), intrusion symptoms (Cluster B), persistent avoidance (Cluster C), negative alterations in cognitions and mood associated with the traumatic events (Cluster D), and hyperarousal (Cluster E). In addition, the duration of the disorder must be more than one month (Cluster F), the disturbance must cause

---

[239] "Exploring the Relationship Between Parkinson's and PTSD." Dr. C. "Possibilities with Parkinson's," Published on Parkinson's News Today, January 10, 2020.

[240] "I Feel Terrorized by the Parkinson's Disease Thief." Dr. C. "Possibilities with Parkinson's," Published on Parkinson's News Today, October 19, 2018.

[241] "The Insular Cortex Dopamine Center and Its Relationship to Parkinson's." Dr. C. "Possibilities with Parkinson's," Published on Parkinson's News Today, October 9, 2020.

clinically significant distress or impairment in social, occupational, or other important areas of functioning (Cluster G), and the *disturbance must not be attributable to the physiological effects of a substance or another medical condition* (Cluster G). The one new diagnostic cluster (Cluster D) in the proposed diagnostic system for PTSD, which was not present in DSM-IV, involves negative alteration in cognition and mood associated with the traumatic event, as evidenced by two or more of seven listed symptoms.[242]

If you are a combat war vet (like me), then the chances are you fit the first criteria (exposure to extreme stress). But one doesn't need combat to meet that criteria. Being told you have PD and dealing with the progression *is* extreme stress.

With PD, there is an added handicap – the malfunctioning second dopamine center. It malfunctions in a way that mimics PTSD, causing many of the symptoms that are diagnostically associated with PTSD. This includes intrusive thoughts, change in cognitive functioning, change in mood, hyperarousal, and significant impairment in functioning. In my case, attribution of PTSD continues to be suggested as a stand-alone clinical diagnosis. It serves as a barrier to quality treatment. The most important part of the PTSD criteria is that the symptoms must not be attributable to an organic malfunction. If the practitioner misses the fact that an organic issue is the main source of the problem, then the result will be poor treatment and poor outcomes.

In my story about the untrained dog crashing through my garden,[243] I mention that the brain places a high emotional

---

[242] Cornelius, Jack R. "Editorial Regarding the New DSM-5 Diagnosis of PTSD in Veterans and Non-veterans." *Journal of depression & anxiety* vol. 2,3 (2013): 139-141. doi:10.4172/2167-1044.1000139

[243] "Loud Emotions Can Be Risky. Here's How to Change Course." Dr. C. "Possibilities with Parkinson's," Published on Parkinson's News Today, August 21, 2020.

value on life threatening situations. It will further enhance the emotive value of those memories. The higher the emotive value, the more likely it is that the memories will become intrusive. This is because the brain is designed to pay attention to memories which have the highest emotion value, those deemed to be most significant to our survival. It is a system that has served our species well over the past millions of years. The problem with atypical non-tremor PD is that it comes with its own version of heightened emotional input due to a faulty second dopamine center. It looks like PTSD, but it is not.

Both extreme trauma and the faulty second dopamine center create heightened emotive input. It can be confusing to both patient and practitioner. If practitioner can take the time to ask the patient about symptoms associated with a faulty second dopamine center, then it may be possible to improve treatment for those PD patients who also have symptoms like PTSD. I propose we develop new diagnostic criteria and add atypical non-tremor PD so that a more accurate diagnosis can be made by practitioners.

Maybe next time I see a neurologist, he won't say, "You don't show a typical PD presentation. And you might have PTSD." Instead, the doctor will say with confidence, "You are a textbook example of atypical non-tremor Parkinson's disease with symptoms that look like PTSD."

A Spectrum Stage Theory for Parkinson's

When I was struggling with health-care providers to arrive at the right diagnosis, I kept wondering, why is Parkinson's so difficult to diagnose?

I asked my favorite neurologist back in 2014, "Has anyone come up with a good theory explaining the large variability in how Parkinson's presents?" He answered, at that time, that there was none.

Other Parkinson's patients have told me, "If you have seen one PD patient, then that's what you've seen." The following figure represents an early version of a new theory to help explain the wide range of clinical features associated with Parkinson's disease:

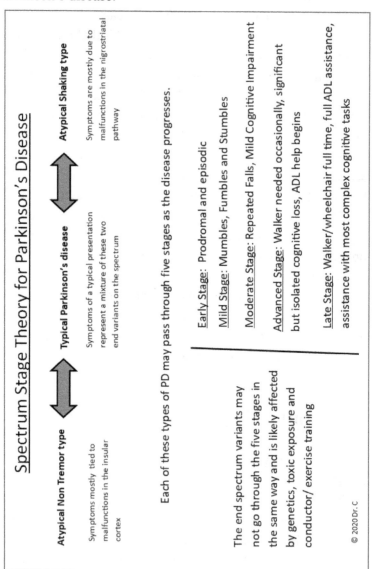

Spectrum Stage Theory for Parkinson's Disease

Atypical Non Tremor type

Symptoms mostly tied to malfunctions in the insular cortex

Typical Parkinson's disease

Symptoms of a typical presentation represent a mixture of these two end variants on the spectrum

Atypical Shaking type

Symptoms are mostly due to malfunctions in the nigrostriatal pathway

Each of these types of PD may pass through five stages as the disease progresses.

Early Stage: Prodromal and episodic

Mild Stage: Mumbles, Fumbles and Stumbles

Moderate Stage: Repeated Falls, Mild Cognitive Impairment

Advanced Stage: Walker needed occasionally, significant but isolated cognitive loss, ADL help begins

Late Stage: Walker/wheelchair full time, full ADL assistance, assistance with most complex cognitive tasks

The end spectrum variants may not go through the five stages in the same way and is likely affected by genetics, toxic exposure and conductor/exercise training

© 2020 Dr. C

The evidence to support the features in this new theory has been presented in earlier columns. Let's review:

1) There is growing evidence that suggests this disorder may be two diseases, one more brain-centered and the other body-centered.[244] BioNews reader comments to my columns suggest many people have non-tremor PD. There is a striking similarity of shared symptoms that readers report that do not necessarily include tremors.

2) There is a second major area in the brain linked to dopamine use called the insular cortex.[245] This second dopamine center is thought to be tied to many of PD nonmotor symptoms.[246] I present as a case study[247] for atypical non-tremor PD – the opposite end in the spectrum from the more obvious shaking PD.

3) The new theory needs a new definition of early-stage PD. Research on prodromal features has been accumulating, pointing us toward a better

---

[244] "Brain Imaging Study Suggests Parkinson's Might Actually Be Two Diseases in One." By Carly Cassella, published on ScienceAlert, September 24, 2020. The study referenced in this article online was first published in the journal Brain: Horsager, Jacob, et al. "Brain-first versus body-first Parkinson's disease: a multimodal imaging case-control study." Brain, Volume 143, Issue 10, October 2020, Pages 3077–3088, https://doi.org/10.1093/brain/awaa238

[245] "The Insular Cortex Dopamine Center and Its Relationship to Parkinson's." Dr. C. "Possibilities with Parkinson's," Published on Parkinson's News Today, October 9, 2020.

[246] "The Default Mode Network: Lies From the Insular Cortex." Dr. C. "Possibilities with Parkinson's," Published on Parkinson's News Today, October 16, 2020.

[247] "My Parkinson's Portrait Is Outside the Classic Criteria." Dr. C. "Possibilities with Parkinson's," Published on Parkinson's News Today, October 2, 2020.

understanding of early PD.[248] Many readers of my columns in Parkinson's News Today report symptoms for 10 to 20 years before final diagnosis of PD.

4) Early intervention with the conductor training and physical exercise may have strong influence on the presentation, management, and progression of PD. It is not only mixtures of the two variants in the spectrum that contributes to a diverse presentation, but also pre-morbid and co-morbid status. Readers report success with physical and mental exercise: If you don't use it, you lose it.

There is no reason to assume that the disease process attacking dopamine neurons would be uniform across the population. Viewing PD as a spectrum between two extreme variants of the disease (influenced by brain/body lifestyles) helps to explain the varied clinical presentation, including why about half of the people diagnosed with PD acquire depression or anxiety only after diagnosis.[249]

Simply put, how you use your brain affects how it functions, especially following trauma or brain disease. The brain is malleable and responds to what we do most with our brains – developing easy to use neural pathways along these well-worn feeling-thought-action paths. Some of the PD variability is likely due to these paths being disrupted by the disease and then being modified as we try to cope (sometimes ineffectually). With this new theory, we can develop brain retraining programs which could mitigate some PD effects.

It all starts with a theory that better describes the way the disease presents. In commentary on the article published by

[248] "It's Time to Redefine Early Stage Parkinson's." Dr. C. "Possibilities with Parkinson's," Published on Parkinson's News Today, October 30, 2020.

[249] "A Fresh Look at Depression and Chronic Illness." Dr. C. "Possibilities with Parkinson's," Published on Parkinson's News Today, July 31, 2020.

Melissa J. Armstrong, M.D., M.Sc., and Michael S. Okun, M.D., "Time for a New Image of Parkinson Disease" in the JAMA Neurology (July 2020),[250] David Blacker, a physician at the Perron Institute for Neurological and Translational Science, offers a refreshingly honest perception:

> What we say as doctors to patients is highly impactful; words need to be chosen carefully and perceptions of illness count. I suspect that mental perception of PD may even influence progression; if a negative, nihilistic image is formed around the time of diagnosis, the self-fulfilling prophecy concept, combined with apathy, could contribute to lack of engagement in physical therapy and mobility, which I suspect accelerates progression.

Dr. Blacker reveals his journey in a most insightful manner in his article, "A Neurologist with Parkinson's Disease."[251] He also states, "I now feel much more confident with the early diagnosis and management and have a much greater insight into the condition."

Another comment on the article of Armstrong and Okun, by Jonny Acheson, a physician at University Hospitals of Leicester,[252] agrees that "a modern image that a person with Parkinson's can look at and relate to, something that says: yes this is me," is needed [my emphasis added].

The Spectrum Stage Theory offers a more complete picture of the disease. However, it is a fledgling construct and should probably be called a "rudimentary theory." It is the coat hanger waiting for the coat. This theory sketch is presented

[250] Armstrong, M.J., and Okun, M.S. "Time for a New Image of Parkinson Disease." *JAMA Neurol.* 2020;77(11): 1345–1346. doi:10.1001/jamaneurol.2020.2412

[251] Blacker, D. "A neurologist with Parkinson's disease." *Practical Neurology* 2020; 20:423-424

[252] Armstrong, M.J., Okun M.S. "Time for a New Image of Parkinson Disease." *JAMA Neurol.* 2020;77(11):1345–1346. doi:10.1001/jamaneurol.2020.2412

for peer review, for discussion among patients and providers, and, most of all, for improvement in our perceptions of the possibilities with Parkinson's.

Afterword: Hope for Humanity

It happened my freshman year in college. My wife and I, just married, were living in a dirt-cheap basement apartment with no windows. In the middle of the night, we abruptly woke to see a glowing, five-foot-diameter ball of sky-blue light in the room. I couldn't see the wall behind it, it did not communicate, and although startled, I wasn't afraid.

I never imagined anything like this would happen. I was a geology major, as down-to-earth as it gets. But this event shook my entire worldview. That was 1971, and this is the first time I've told the story of when an Angel visited.

I wanted so much to discredit the event; like Charles Dickens' character Scrooge observed, it might have been just "an undigested bit of beef." But my wife witnessed it with me. A blue light appeared in a windowless room. We weren't using mind-altering substances. We weren't reading, talking about, or thinking about such an event in any way that might indicate suggestibility. It just happened, and nothing I could say or do would change that.

It came down to a choice: I had to accept the event or accept that my wife and I had a simultaneous delusion, and we were both crazy. When an Angel visits, it's hard to accept.

Moments after the blue light disappeared, I turned to my wife and asked, "What was that?"

"That was for you," she responded.

Like Paul on the road to Damascus, it was a rebirth moment. I was awakened to the possibility of the intangible, of real phenomena that existed beyond the rational and scientific realms. After the encounter, I was given a new way of seeing the world, a deeper sense of the interconnectedness of everything. People looked different, and conversations changed. When shaking someone's hand, interconnected patterns unfolded before me, like Christopher Walken's character in *The Dead Zone* when he touches people and sees their life events. When an Angel visits, it offers information to be utilized.

That same year, my sister died in a car crash at age 19. She was my closest sibling, and people often thought of us as twins. My heart was broken, and I sobbed for days. Seeking to console me, my wife said, "Maybe you can talk to her to say goodbye."

Wiping the tears, I replied, "That would be great, but impossible. She is dead, returned to dust, gone forever."

The tears returned. My wife said, "She is a spirit now but not gone. Maybe there is a way to reach out through that beyond what we know."

She told me I needed to find a tunnel of light in my mind. Once I found a tunnel, I needed to walk through it. There was a chance I would be able to talk to my sister on the other side of the tunnel.

If the blue-light event hadn't just happened, I would've thought all of this to be crazy, supernatural hogwash. If my sister hadn't died, I would've lacked the motivation to try such a thing. If it had been anyone else guiding me, I wouldn't have trusted them. The stars were aligned. I found the tunnel.

Suddenly, I was outside my body looking down on myself. I didn't expect that to happen – I was looking for my sister. Shocked, I heard myself say, "I don't want to be here." In an instant, I was back in my body telling my wife that an out-of-body-experience had just happened.

These events left me with three new skills, and I felt called to learn all I could while staying balanced with my love of science. The first was empathic connection with others that yielded a short burst of interconnected patterns from the person I touched. The second was my ability to disconnect the self from this empathic flow while still being an observer – to get out of the way so that the empathic information could be experienced more accurately. Thirdly, I concluded that the process of thinking like a scientist needed to be applied to these observable phenomena across multiple settings. After an Angel visits, new possibilities emerge.

I spent the next 20 years honing my skills in holding together this empathic space for others while advancing my skills as a scientist. Every week, some encounter strengthened my internal dialog that "this is really amazing," which gradually morphed into, "Wow, I am really amazing." It was not where I needed to take myself.

Then, while cycling for 20 miles, which was my daily exercise, I was hit by a car. Everything was taken away; I couldn't sense anyone anymore. I was no longer amazing. From a medical standpoint, I suffered no serious injuries and was released from the ER within hours of the accident. This was before concussions and mild traumatic brain injuries made headlines in the context of athletic injuries. Suffering from a mild traumatic brain injury and not realizing it, combined with other medical issues not yet diagnosed, my life fell apart. We lost everything.

I still held on to that call of finding the balance between science and empathic space. I pursued a Ph.D., but things didn't start smoothly. My first semester left me with a future unknown and the dread of failure. For days, I remained curled up in a fetal position facing a darkness I had never seen before. I saw no way out.

Then I heard a voice say to me as clearly as if someone were in the chair next to me, "Get up and go for a walk in the park." I was compelled to do just that. Walking through the sanctuary of the park, I saw a bright ball of light illuminating a tree by the lake, conveying the message, "God loves you.

Continue this sacred path and all will be fine. Go in peace."

At the edge of the lake, I dropped to my knees in awe and humble gratitude. When I stood, I noticed the water was filled with tightly packed rainbow trout, wiggling ever so slightly, and causing waves of iridescence that seemed magical. When an Angel visits, darkness disappears.

Heartened by this experience, I returned to my studies. For my doctorate, I examined the empathic space that skilled healers have described, and what people have said about those experiences with healers. Soon after completing my dissertation, I began to develop a scientific way of describing this special relationship.

I define compassion as the empathy to identify suffering plus the wisdom to do something about reducing it. This is what healers do, and what is often experienced by the people who go to them.

Further, I define empathy as having the following characteristics: receipt of information, reflection on that information, mutuality, proper intent, and a developmental aspect. This special relationship with others has a specific purpose: to help people reduce suffering in their lives. I called it the "healing relationship."

As empathy plus wisdom, compassion is at the heart of the healing relationship and frames proper intent for practicing it. This was something that fit my calling, the sacred events of my life, and the demands of the scientist. It fit my new role of mystic scientist. My insights into the healing relationship came from these sacred life experiences, along with academic study and the practice of healing.

The main elements of the healing relationship are a facilitating agent, someone seeking healing, and a witness. How the healing process is understood by all participants and the intent that frames the process shape the experience. The agent can be someone who facilitates healing, a sacred place where healing occurs, a healing in connection with a near-death experience, a miraculous and spontaneous remission of a disease, or a placebo effect. They all have common features found in the healing relationship. The witness guards the before and after documentation, and it is best if they are present at the healing event. The entire process, if framed within the proper intent of compassion, is often deemed sacred.

After a lifetime of investigation, I have developed a basic working definition of the healing relationship. It is a special relationship a person can enter while directly experiencing a moment of well-being, accompanied by a wellness map showing how to discover more well-being moments. The wellness map is personal to each individual and revealed rather than taught.

Healing occurs within this relationship as a reduction of suffering and often is accompanied by a reduction in physical symptoms that are blocking well-being moments from occurring. It is the relationship that skilled healers have been entering into for millennia. We have forgotten the nature of the healing relationship, and in our amnesia, we mistake it for other types of relationships. In those mistakes and misunderstandings lies the potential for misuse and abuse.

The Beatles sang, "All you need is love," which became the theme of the counterculture movement. I think so much suffering is connected to the unquestioned love of a dogma, a country, or a possessive love of another. If asked to love my enemy, is it brotherly love, like comrades in arms? Should it be like love for family, for my mother or father, or how I love my children? Maybe it's the love associated with "I love days like this" or "I love my job."

It's easy to see all the pain and misery caused in the name of love. I wouldn't offer this chaos and confusion to my worst enemy. Instead, I'd gladly offer the healing relationship. Perhaps if we can understand the nature of the healing relationship, we can eliminate some of the confusion, decrease the suffering, and help save humanity from itself.

The concept of the healing relationship as growth that fosters relationship is not new. What is new is to have a phenomenological construct that can be used as a foundation for further scientific research. I don't know how this special relationship happens or whether there are special conditions that make the healing relationship more likely to occur. The difficulty lies in educating others about construct definition so that research may explore the how, when, where, and why. People bring to the idea of a healing relationship their current understanding of human relationships. There is a limit to how personal knowledge can be used for understanding the healing relationship, which is experiential.

I also don't know if the experience of the healing relationship is similar across a large portion of the population. What I do know is that after many years of research, writing, and exploration of the idea, a foundation of understanding now exists for further study.

It was a calling that I had to follow. Along the way, I traveled some wrong paths, and some dark ones, and I met resistance. At other times, I found shared understanding. Looking back, everything seems to have fit the calling, even if I couldn't see it at the time. Above all, I have never wavered in the belief that my calling has been worthwhile and helpful to many.

I look forward to someone picking up the baton of healing relationship research. It will be exciting to see an application of the evidence that exists, and evidence yet to be discovered, to the remaining questions about the healing relationship.

When an Angel visits and shows you your calling, stick with it and be sure to say thank you, even if it's half a century later.

About Atmosphere Press

Atmosphere Press is an independent, full-service publisher for excellent books in all genres and for all audiences. Learn more about what we do at atmospherepress.com.

We encourage you to check out some of Atmosphere's latest releases, which are available at Amazon.com and via order from your local bookstore:

Convergence: The Interconnection of Extraordinary Experiences, by Barbara Mango, Ph.D., and Lynn Miller, MS

One Warrior to Another: A Vietnam Combat Veteran's Reflection, by Richard Cleaves

Emotional Liberation: Life Beyond Triggers and Trauma, by GuruMeher Khalsa

License to Learn: Elevating Discomfort in Service of Lifelong Learning, by Anna Switzer, Ph.D.

Sex—Interrupted: Igniting Intimacy While Living With Illness or Disability, by Iris Zink and Jenny Palter

Waking Up Marriage: Finding Truth Inside Your Partnership, by Bill O'Herron

An Ambiguous Grief, by Dominique Hunter

My Take on All Fifty States: An Unexpected Quest to See 'Em All, by Jim Ford

Chasing the Dragon's Tail: Finding Passion in Your Purpose, by Craig Fullerton

About the Author

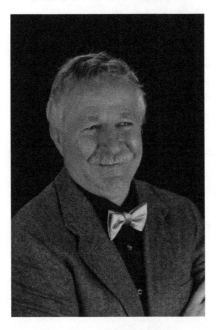

"Dr. C" is the non-de-plume for W. David Hoisington. He earned his Ph. D. in rehabilitation counselling from Syracuse University where he studied advanced levels of empathy. Empathy, along with understanding of how the brain functions, were fundamental to providing quality rehabilitation plans for those with cerebral neurologic trauma – the focus of his clinical practice. He was exposed to Agent Orange resulting in Parkinson's disease which, through a twist of fate, led him to writing a weekly column on his experiences with PD. The essays in this book combine empathy and brain functions to address the disease in a new, more hopeful, way.

CPSIA information can be obtained
at www.ICGtesting.com
Printed in the USA
LVHW041006080621
689682LV00005B/238

9 781637 528662